Health professions and the state in Europe

D0264558

Governments throughout the world are increasingly concerned with the costs and quality of health care. Health professionals internationally are facing major changes and are re-examining both their organizational and skill base in order to sustain their services to sponsors and clients. Focusing on the theme of change, *Health Professions and the State in Europe* explores the responses to these challenges across the shifting socio-political map of Europe.

The editors and contributors, all established authorities in their field, develop analytical models to explain and illuminate the changing character of professions, as influenced by governments and other agencies, with particular reference to the health arena. They then consider the specific relationship between health professions and the state in Britain and a number of other European countries – Spain, Belgium, the Netherlands, Scandinavia and the Czech Republic. Topical issues of international and comparative relevance are covered, such as the impact on the health professions of market policies, performance and quality measures, and challenges to professional monopolies and expertise.

Health Professions and the State in Europe presents an overview of the current situation in eight European countries. As such it enhances our understanding of the interplay between health professions and the state in different national contexts in relation to a wide range of health professions, including nursing, midwifery and medicine. It will be of special relevance to students, teachers and professionals with interests in health policy, social policy and medical sociology.

Terry Johnson is Professor of Sociology at the University of Leicester. **Gerry Larkin** is Professor of the Sociology of Health and Illness at Sheffield Hallam University. **Mike Saks** is Professor and Head of the School of Health and Life Sciences at De Montfort University, Leicester.

Health professions and the state in Europe

Edited by Terry Johnson, Gerry Larkin and Mike Saks

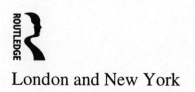

London and New York

First published 1995
by Routledge
11 New Fetter Lane, London EC4P 4EE

Simultaneously published in the USA and Canada
by Routledge
29 West 35th Street, New York, NY 10001

© 1995 Terry Johnson, Gerry Larkin and Mike Saks, selection and editorial matter; the chapters, the contributors.

Typeset in Times by LaserScript, Mitcham, Surrey
Printed and bound in Great Britain by
TJ Press (Padstow) Ltd, Padstow, Cornwall

All rights reserved. No part of this book may be reprinted or reproduced or utilized in any form or by any electronic, mechanical, or other means, now known or hereafter invented, including photocopying and recording, or in any information storage or retrieval system, without permission in writing from the publishers.

British Library Cataloguing in Publication Data
A catalogue record for this book is available from the British Library

Library of Congress Cataloging in Publication Data
A catalog record for this book has been requested

ISBN 0–415–10630–3 (hbk)
ISBN 0–415–10631–1 (pbk)

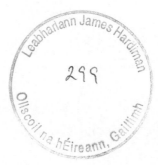
Leabharlann James Hardiman
Ollscoil na hÉireann, Gaillimh
299

Contents

Contributors

EDITORS

Professor Terry Johnson is a member of the Department of Sociology at the University of Leicester. He has gained an international reputation from his seminal book *Professions and Power* (Macmillan 1972) which has been reinforced by subsequent work. His latest publications include a co-edited volume with Mike Gane entitled *Foucault's New Domains* (Routledge 1993).

Professor Gerry Larkin is a member of the School of Health and Community Studies at Sheffield Hallam University. His research interests cover the social history of health care and the sociology of the professions. He has published extensively on the historical and contemporary development of health professions. He is the author of the well-regarded book *Occupational Monopoly and Modern Medicine* (Tavistock 1983).

Professor Mike Saks is Head of the School of Health and Life Sciences at De Montfort University, Leicester. He is best known for his work on professions and health care. His most important recent publications include an edited collection on *Alternative Medicine in Britain* (Clarendon Press 1992) and *Professions and the Public Interest: Medical Power, Altruism and Alternative Medicine* (Routledge 1994).

CONTRIBUTORS

Professor Andy Alaszewski is Director of the Institute of Health Studies at the University of Hull.

Professor Judith Allsop holds a chair in Health Policy at South Bank University.

Dr Mike Dent is a member of the School of Social Sciences at Staffordshire University.

Dr Vibeke Erichsen is based at the Norwegian Research Centre of Organization and Management at the University of Bergen in Norway.

Professor Alena Heitlinger is a member of the Department of Sociology at Trent University, Ontario in Canada.

Leonie van der Hulst is a sociologist who is actively involved in midwifery in the Netherlands.

Professor Terry Johnson is a member of the Department of Sociology at the University of Leicester.

Professor Gerry Larkin holds a chair in the Sociology of Health and Illness at Sheffield Hallam University.

Professor Donald Light is Professor of Comparative Health Care Systems at the University of Medicine and Dentistry of New Jersey in the United States.

Professor Elianne Riska is a member of the Department of Sociology at the Åbo Academi University in Finland.

Dr Josep Rodríguez is a member of the Department of Sociology at the University of Barcelona in Spain.

Professor Mike Saks is Head of the School of Health and Life Sciences at De Montfort University, Leicester.

Dr Rita Schepers is a member of the Department of Health Care Policy and Management at the Erasmus University, Rotterdam, in the Netherlands.

Professor Meg Stacey is Emeritus Professor of Sociology at the University of Warwick.

Edwin van Teijlingen is based at the Centre for HIV/AIDS and Drug Studies at the City Hospital in Edinburgh in Scotland.

Katarina Wegar is a member of the Department of Sociology at Colorado College in the United States.

Acknowledgements

The editors wish to express their appreciation to all of the authors for their contributions and for the most helpful way in which they responded to queries throughout the production of this volume. Thanks are also due to Anita Bishop who assisted with the typing of the manuscript.

Introduction

Terry Johnson, Gerry Larkin and Mike Saks

The contributions to this edited collection are based on a number of the many papers first presented at the International Sociological Association conference on Professions in Transition, held in Leicester in April 1992. The original theme of the conference reflected the widespread view amongst academics that an accumulating range of changes occurring on an international scale necessitated a review of the professions. In selecting the papers for this volume the editors have continued the focus on the theme of change, both in conceptual and analytical terms and through illustrations of the developing nature and role of particular professions in a variety of national contexts. The international flavour of the volume in this latter respect is encapsulated in the fact that it includes contributions from leading authors on the professions from eight different countries, spanning Britain, Europe and North America.

While professions in general have been involved in many major transitions in recent decades, this has arguably nowhere been more apparent than in the field of health care. This has further guided the selection of papers, as has an awareness that a wider review of sociological and historical perspectives on professions can assist in understanding specific areas of change. Amongst the ranks of health professions new occupations and reformed segments from more established occupational groups constantly emerge, reshaping relationships within the division of labour. In addition, apparently unchallenged professions are perpetually compelled to re-examine their organizational and skill base to sustain their services to sponsors and clients. The processes of resistance and change within and between professions therefore need to be documented and understood, but within a further context of adjustments in previous relationships with the state and other major sponsoring agencies and purchasing bodies.

Pressures for reflection and change often emanate from forces outside of the immediate professional field, and in health care these have globally been very significant. Such pressures have particularly originated in recent decades from fundamental policy changes by governments in the broad area of welfare, and sometimes more profoundly still in basic alterations of the character of the state itself. The case of policy change within established frameworks of government can be illustrated with reference to the various experiments with *laissez-faire* approaches through the 1980s. These are linked to perceived fiscal and economic crises in democratic capitalist states, and are evident in health policy through a near universal preoccupation with cost-containment. Examples of shifts in the nature of the state cover not only the growing regulation of once sovereign states through their inclusion in complexes of international regulation – as in the European Community – but also transformations in the ideology and administration of individual states. In this respect, the world has recently witnessed the dissolution of a number of regimes of a fascist and communist persuasion. Changes of this magnitude have presented both radical dilemmas and new opportunities for professions nurtured in the image and values of the previous regime. Irrespective of the source of shifts in the direction of state policy, a comparative international focus is instructive. This has influenced the choice of contents here, which centres on the European context in which such transformations affecting the health professions are well exemplified.

In pursuing the theme of transition in relation to the health professions in Europe, the book is divided into three main sections. The first part of the book begins by highlighting some of the key analytical issues involved in understanding the interplay between professions and the state, with reference to the health arena. The next part of the text continues the state–professions theme with reference to illustrations drawn from the medical profession and other health professional groups in Britain. It covers such areas as the historical relationship between health professions and the state, the recently introduced internal market in health care, community care, peer review and quality assurance, the interface between orthodox and unorthodox medicine, and professional regulation in the shifting socio-political environment in Britain. The final part broadens the international scope of the volume by examining the relationship between health professions and the state in a number of other countries in Europe – including Spain, Belgium, the Netherlands, Sweden, Finland, Norway and the Czech Republic. This section again considers professional groups like nursing and midwifery as well as medicine and encapsulates the main strand of the book – the changing relationship between the state and the professions in health care.

Moving on to a more detailed breakdown of the contents in each section, the two orientational chapters contained in Part I of the book raise general issues bearing on the changing relationship between the modern state and the professions. Following an exploration of the more important sociological contributions to this theme, Terry Johnson in chapter 1 argues that Michel Foucault's concept of governmentality provides a novel and more fruitful approach, by rejecting conventional theories which counterpose professions and the state and focusing on the processes of government. In chapter 2 Donald Light suggests that the concept of countervailing powers best conceptualizes the political processes involved in health policy outcomes.

Turning to the consideration of Britain in Part II of the volume, in chapter 3 Gerry Larkin focuses on the way in which the governing process in the twentieth century has led to the formation and transformation of a medico-bureaucratic network that moulds the changing relationship between the state and health professions, as well as between the health professions themselves. In chapter 4

Andy Alaszewski compares the medical profession with the professions of nursing and social work in order to suggest that recent government reforms in Britain have created a series of internal markets for professional services. In chapter 5 Judith Allsop examines changes in general practice over the past ten years, in the context of policy changes which have emphasized both quasi-market principles and increased state control. The impact of competitive forces and governmental regulation on professional autonomy are considered in terms of its possible enhancement and partial erosion in these changing circumstances. In chapter 6 Mike Dent further considers government-sponsored internal market policies, but with reference to hospital doctors and the development of medical audit and quality assurance reviews. These are discussed in both their British and earlier American applications, with a focus on the tensions between organizational and professional forms of control. In chapter 7 Mike Saks broadens the consideration of professional control to consider whether the strong link between orthodox medicine and the state is to the public benefit. The development of acupuncture is explored to suggest that the medical profession, even when revising its policies towards alternative therapies, consolidates its own position. Finally, in chapter 8 of this section Meg Stacey explores the General Medical Council's policies of regulating competition in the professional market from overseas and European qualified doctors. Both change and continuity in the General Medical Council are examined as its focus shifts from post-imperial to European dimensions of professional regulation.

Part III of the book moves on to consider the relationship between health professions and the state in continental Europe. In chapter 9, Josep Rodríguez assesses the impact of democratization and the creation of a dominant public health care system on the medical profession in Spain. It is argued that the implementation of these reforms has increased the degree of proletarianization of the medical profession – a trend that is now becoming even more accentuated in the private health sector, with the growing involvement of large corporations. Rita Schepers observes in chapter 10 that the recent activities of the government and the private sickness funds in the medical market have also brought about changes in the position of Belgian doctors, although it is as yet unclear whether the power and autonomy of the medical profession is in real decline. Such power and autonomy are typically greater than that possessed by the subordinated midwives in the industrialized world. However, Edwin van Teijlingen and Leonie van der Hulst claim in chapter 11 that the state in the Netherlands has granted midwifery more independence from the medical profession than in either Britain or the United States, partly because of the greater emphasis on state regulation of the social obligations of individual professions in continental Europe. But if this underlines the significance of the state in shaping the jurisdiction of the health professions, so too does chapter 12 by Vibeke Erichsen, who argues that the Scandinavian countries fit neither the predominant Anglo-American practitioner-driven nor the classic European state-driven models of professionalization. Rather, she suggests that the process of medical professionalization in Sweden and Norway at least has been based on a close interdependent relationship between doctors and state bureaucracies. Elianne Riska and Katarina Wegar in chapter 13 add a further dimension to the discussion of the state–profession interface in focusing on the gender balance in the medical profession in Norway and Finland. This has become an increasingly important issue as the state has shifted resources to primary care where it is argued women doctors are more strongly represented because of their perceived mastery of work involving the emotions. The section and the book conclude with chapter 14 by Alena Heitlinger which illuminates the central theme of changing state–profession relationships in Europe by examining the position of medicine and nursing in the new post-communist Czech Republic, following the break-up of longstanding party control.

Readers of this book may wish to explore particular national case studies or theoretical and comparative issues relating to health professions and the state in Europe. However, while the text may be read for immediate points of interest, it has also been constructed to hang together as a whole. At the same time, the authors of each chapter have developed their own particular analyses. The editors consider that the associated variation in style and approach contributes to the richness of this volume and its value to those concerned with professions, health care and the state in both national and international settings.

Part I

Professions and the state: theoretical issues

1 Governmentality and the institutionalization of expertise

Terry Johnson

What is happening to the professions? In both Europe and the United States there exists the growing certainty that those occupations that established such high-status, independent and privileged locations in the division of labour from the mid-nineteenth century onwards are undergoing fundamental change. In Britain, the dominant image of the professional as a sole, male practitioner, personally and independently servicing individual clients, has, in the second half of the twentieth century, gradually disintegrated in the face of a reality of increasingly diverse work locations, many of them bureaucratic in character. Also, in recent years, this gradual transformation has been quickened by the 'deregulation' policies of the government; policies which have their parallels on the Continent and in the United States.

The popular image of the professions as made up of independent, solo practitioners was, for a considerable period, remarkably resistant to the changing realities of the division of labour, transformed by such processes as the rise of the large-scale, technological hospital; the growth of professional bureaucracies of lawyers and accountants organizationally rooted in the myth of partnership; the incorporation of new and old professions into burgeoning state agencies; and the world-wide spread of multinational business firms maintaining their own corps of professional employees.

These processes of transformation are today well established, and the number of professionals practising in novel work sites far outnumber those remaining in traditional locations. While there is general agreement in the sociological literature about the scope of these changes, there is little agreement about their consequences and, more important for us, we still await a generally accepted perspective explaining the significance of these changes which we all observe. The current need for theoretical advance is, however, hindered by a conception of expertise which remains too closely tied to the professions' own view of themselves. In particular we are blinkered by a misconception of the relationship between the professions and the state; a relationship which British professionals characteristically view as the primary threat to their independence.

The object of this chapter will be to argue that the institutionalization of expertise in the form of the professions in the modern world has been integral to what Foucault (1979) calls governmentality. Briefly, Foucault's concept of government rejects the notion of the state as a coherent, calculating subject whose political power grows in concert with its interventions into civil society. Rather, the state is viewed as an ensemble of institutions, procedures, tactics, calculations, knowledges and technologies, which together comprise the particular form that government has taken; the outcome of governing.

FOUCAULT AND GOVERNMENTALITY

According to Foucault, governmentality is a novel capacity for governing that gradually emerged in Europe from the sixteenth century onwards in association with the invention, operationalization and institutionalization of specific knowledges, disciplines, tactics and technologies. The period from the sixteenth until the eighteenth century was, he argues, notable for the appearance throughout Europe of a series of treatises on government: on the government of the soul and the self; on the government of children within the family; on the government of the state (Foucault 1979: 5–9). This rethinking of the various forms of governance was associated both with the early formation of the great territorial, administrative states and colonial empires, and with the disruptions of spiritual rule associated with the reformation and counter-reformation. Together, these discourses on government were precursors of the disciplines of morality, economics and politics.

While the latter initially focused on juridical conceptions of sovereignty, Foucault (1979: 12) identifies a revolutionary break with the Machiavellian assumption that the power of the prince was best deployed in securing sovereignty, to the view that governing was no more than the 'right disposition of things' leading to the 'common welfare and salvation of all'. This novel discourse which began to conceive of popular obedience to the law as the sole source of legitimate rule (that is to say, sovereignty and law were rendered synonymous) also made it possible to identify – in the capacity to make 'dispositions of things' – the means of governing, those tactics and knowledges developed in order to regulate territories and populations. Statistics, for example, revealed that populations had their own regularities; such as rates of death, disease and cycles of scarcity. These were regularities of structure irreducible to the family as the object of rule. Thus, claims Foucault (1979: 13–16), the art of government gave way to a science of government.

> It was thanks to the perception of the specific problems of population, related to the isolation of that area of reality that we call the economy, that the problem of government finally came to be thought, reflected and calculated outside the juridical framework of sovereignty.
>
> (1979: 16)

That form of government which came to have population as its object of rule, and political economy as its principal form of knowledge, was an ensemble of institutions, procedures, analyses, calculations, reflections and tactics that constituted *governmentality*, a 'very specific albeit complex form of power' (1979: 19); the form of government that came to characterize modernity.

What we can add to – or derive from – Foucault's analysis is that in the course of the eighteenth and particularly the nineteenth centuries expertise – the social organization of these emergent disciplines – became integral to this process of governmentality. That is to say, that during this period expertise became as much a condition for the exercise of political power as did the formal bureaucratic apparatus we often, mistakenly, identify as constituting the state (see Miller and Rose 1990). In short, expertise, as it became increasingly institutionalized in its professional form, became part of the process of governing.

In developing this argument, the chapter has two goals. The first is to use the insights inherent in Foucault's concept of governmentality to open up a new domain of Foucauldian analysis, the institutionalization of expertise. In achieving this objective we hope to displace the terms of a long-standing controversy in the sociology of the professions regarding the source and degree of professional autonomy in the face of state intervention. The autonomy/intervention controversy in the sociology of the professions arises, it will be argued, only insofar as the relationship between state and professions is misconceived as one existing between two subjects.

FREIDSON AND FOUCAULT: TWO VIEWS OF THE STATE

The dominant conception of the state/profession relationship found in the sociological literature is a systematic source of serious dispute and controversy. It generates argument about the nature and degree of autonomy enjoyed by professional practitioners (Freidson 1973; Haug 1973; Light and Levine 1988); the degree of state intervention into or state control of professional practice (Lewis and Maude 1952; Navarro 1976; Wright 1978); the extent to which the professions enjoy a post-industrial dominance as an élite (Bell 1960); and the degree to which they are increasingly subordinated to the control of corporate capital and are consequently undergoing a process of proletarianization (Oppenheimer 1973; Derber 1982; McKinlay and Stoeckle 1988).

While such disputes, insofar as they focus on the profession/state relationship, may be exacerbated by the import of exogenous values into the analysis, there is little doubt that a significant source of such disagreement (and, one might add, mutual incomprehension) is the pervasive conception of state/profession as a relationship between preconstituted, coherent, calculating political subjects; one intervening, the other seeking autonomy. While the professions are seen as acting to maximize autonomy, the state is presented as continuously extending its apparatuses of control throughout society, including over the professions.

This dominant and conventional view of the relationship has been one-dimensional; that is, comprising only one set of alternatives – externally imposed control or internally generated autonomy. Eliot Freidson was undoubtedly the first sociologist to provide a more systematic and sophisticated view of the relationship. In *Profession of Medicine* Freidson (1970) directly and effectively confronted the issue: how is it possible to acknowledge the extent to which a profession is subject to state regulation, even state control, while at the same time retaining the view that such occupations are characterized by their autonomy or independence? Freidson's answer was simple, but seminal.

Medicine, he argued, like other professions, emerged by the 'grace of power-ful protectors' (Freidson 1970: xii) and it was from such a protected 'shelter' in the nineteenth century that it was able to achieve autonomy, both from the ideological dominance of such protective élites and, subsequently, from the constraining effects of all external evaluation including that exercised by govern-ments. Freidson posed the question: Can an occupation be truly autonomous, a profession free, when it must submit to the protective custody of the state (1970: 24)? He answered that while a profession may be entirely subordinated to the state when it comes to the 'social and economic organisation of work', never-theless, modern states, whatever their ideological leanings, 'uniformly' leave in the hands of professions control over the *technical* aspect of their work (1970: 24). In the United States, for example, doctors retain control over the 'quality and the terms of medical practice' (1970: 33). In Britain the British Medical Asso-ciation controls 'the determination of the technical standards of medical work, and seems to have the strongest voice in determining what is ethical and un-ethical' (1970: 39). State intervention does not, Freidson suggested, undermine the autonomy of technical judgement so much as establish the social or moral premises on which the judgement of illness is based (1970: 43). The technical aspect of medical work remains immune from external and, therefore, 'pro-fessionally intolerable' evaluation. Thus Freidson says,

> so long as a profession is free of the technical evaluation and control of other occupations in the division of labour, its lack of ultimate freedom from the state, and even its lack of control over the socio-economic terms of work do not significantly change its *essential character as profession.*
>
> (1970: 25; original emphasis)

In short, within the protected socio-political environment or 'shelter' provided by the state a profession may be secured from serious, 'alternative' practitioner competition, while wielding independent power sufficient to control virtually all technical 'facets of its work'. For Freidson, then, autonomy of technique is what defines a profession as well as its relationship with the state. Freidson solved his initial problem, therefore, by way of the claim that the automony of a profession depended on its dependence on the state. The ensuing paradox is resolved once we distinguish between the types of autonomy (technical as against socio-economic) and forms of dependence (absolute and relative). Freidson was in effect countering the powerful rhetoric of practising professionals who claimed a tradition of gentlemanly independence, and continued to fight for absolute autonomy from the encroachments of the 'interventionist' state. Freidson seemed to be recognizing a postwar reality by accepting that the state increasingly held the professions in an intimate socio-economic embrace while, at the same time, providing the professions with a theoretical underpinning for their claim of independence; the autonomy of technical evaluation.

Despite his achievement, Freidson remained tied to a conception of the state as an external, calculating subject; a state that provides 'shelter', exerts control over the socio-economic terms of professional work, leaves matters of technical evaluation in the hands of professionals. It is this conception which ultimately leads to an incoherence in Freidson's position; an incoherence that Foucault's conception of governmentality allows us to overcome. The general relevance of Foucault for this issue is best approached by way of his historiography; that is to say, from his rejection of any conception of history as the unfolding of an essence, or as a search for origins.

As is illustrated by Freidson himself, there is a strong tradition in sociology wedded to the belief that an occupation has the potential to become a profession only when it is heir to a body of esoteric knowledge (Parsons 1949; Barber 1963). In short, a process of professionalization – towards the end-state of professionalism in which an occupation controls its own destiny – is essentially a product of this knowledge potential. In the story of professionalization as an historical process, state intervention is often viewed as a major impediment, explaining why certain occupations fail to attain the full flowering of professionalism. The part played by technique in Freidson's concept of autonomy has an affinity with the conception of professionalization as the unfolding of an essence, knowledge.

In an associated search for origins, students of the professions have normally identified state intervention as a process synonymous with the decline of *laissez-faire*, the mythic separation of state and society during the early nineteenth century. Starting from such a point the history of medicine in Britain, for example, becomes a process of increasing state intervention, leading inexorably to the foundation of the National Health Service. It is a history with only two possible outcomes, autonomy or intervention. Foucault would reject any attempt to present these competing accounts, professionalization or state intervention, as adequate histories. Rather they constitute inadmissible alternatives to history; inadmissible insofar as they are merely the realization of preconstituted essences; an evolution foretold in its origins.

From a Foucauldian perspective a history of the professions becomes one part of the transformation of power associated with governmentality, as 'the disposition of things'. The rapid crystallization of expertise and the establishment of professional associations in the nineteenth century was directly linked to the problems of governmentality – including the classification and surveillance of populations, the normalization of the subject-citizen and the discipline of the aberrant subject. The establishment of the jurisdictions of professions like medicine, psychiatry, law and accountancy, were all consequent on problems of government and, as such, were, from the beginning of the nineteenth century at least, the product of government programmes and policies. Far from emerging autonomously in a period of separation between state and society, the professions were part of the process of state formation.

It follows that equally important for a Foucauldian view of the state/profession relationship is his conception of power as a social relation of tension rather than the attribute of a subject. Given such a conception, power can never be reduced to an act of domination or non-reciprocal intervention. In short, according to Foucault, the relationship of power peculiar to modern liberal democracies emerged with the shift from divine to popular legitimacy. That is to say, in the modern era the legitimate political power has resided in the obedience of subjects, and it is Foucault's central concern with the formation of the obedient subject that explains his focus on the role of discipline (that is, disciplines/ knowledges) in his analysis of modernity. Along with Weber he argues that the outcome of such power is not characteristically domination but the probability that the normalized subject will habitually obey. It is the obedience of the subject-citizen that reproduces the legitimacy of power in the modern liberal-democratic state. Consequently, the actions of subjects; the self, the body, become the objects of new knowledges, new disciplines and technologies which are, in turn, the products of expertise.

The concern with governing is, then, crucially linked to the process of what Foucault calls normalization; the institutionalization of those disciplines/ knowledges that prepare the ground for the reproduction of the normalized, self-regulating subject. Foucault's conception of governmentality focuses our attention on the mechanisms through which the political programmes and objectives of governments have been aligned to the personal and collective conduct of subjects. Governmentality is, in short, all those procedures, techniques, mechanisms, institutions and knowledges that, as an ensemble, empower these political programmes. Most important for our argument is that expertise was crucial to the development of such an ensemble, and that the modern professions were the institutionalized form that such expertise took.

The professions have, then, developed in association with the process of governmentality. To put it another way, the modern professions emerged as part of that apparatus that constitutes the state. The revisionist history of the mental asylum in Britain – influenced by Foucault's *Madness and Civilization* (1973) – is particularly instructive here. First, it has undermined the essentialist view that the building of the asylums was a necessary response to the individual patho-logies of an increasingly anomic, urban, industrial environment. Also it has questioned the view that the medical profession was the obvious and only source of expertise available to staff in the asylums. What has become clear is that the expert classification of the mad, and the emergent typologies of madness, were integral to government policies associated with the problem of pauperism, and that the medical mad-doctor gained official recognition in the role of psychiatric expert only after a struggle with other occupations, as well as resistance from the legislature (Scull 1979). Such an analysis suggests that the emergence of psy-chiatry as a professional specialism was a product of government policy, and that, like the asylum itself, psychiatry emerged as part of that ensemble of disciplines, techniques, tactics and procedures that we now refer to as the state.

The state is not here conceived of as some external, conditioning environment of government. Rather, the state is the outcome of governing; its institutionalized residue, so to speak. It also follows that those procedures and technologies, forms of classification and notation that, in part, embody the state are embedded both in those formal bureaucratic organs that we normally identify as the state apparatus and in the agents of institutionalized expertise, the professions. In short, the state, as the particular form that government has taken in the modern world, includes expertise, or the professions. The duality, profession/state, is eliminated.

To return to Freidson, the continued commitment to such dualism in his work inhibits our capacity to think an empirical reality in which these two realms of activity are inseparable. For example, the crux of Freidson's argument – the autonomy of technique – is rendered vulnerable once we admit that technicality is not the product of colleague discourse alone. In all cases, the technicalities of expert practice entail various combinations of cognitive and normative elements. Some of these are a product of colleague endorsement, while others emerge in the realm of public opinion or originate in official programmes or policies. If it is recognized that technicality is the product of public, professional and official discourse, then in what sense does the profession/state dualism retain meaning? In medicine, even in the determination of such basic categories as 'life' and 'death', where one might expect the technicality of expertise to reign supreme, both public and official discourses are currently very influential and even account, in part at least, for the types of indicators used by medical practitioners. To quote Freidson (1970) again: 'To understand the state of the socially constructed universe at any given time, or its change over time, one must understand the social organization that permits the definers to do their defining'.

If we apply this injunction to the medical profession we are forced to conclude that any attempt radically to separate professional experts from official definers is misconceived, and that in effect doctors are themselves intimately involved in generating official definitions of reality. There is a real sense in which in overseeing established definitions of illness, the profession *is* the state. The privileged place of medical definers in the social order is that they are part of an official realm of discourse. Because expertise is in this sense inseparable from those processes we call the state, it also follows that at this point the medical experts become immune from state control. The expert is not sheltered by an environing state, but shares in the autonomy of the state.

If this conclusion is accepted then it further suggests that the duality, state/profession, functions conceptually to conceal the integrated nature of such processes – the extent to which professionalization and state formation have been different aspects, or profiles, of a single social phenomenon in the modern world. The success of medical professionals in constructing a social reality with universal validity is a consequence of their official recognition as experts. The point at which technical autonomy is established is the very same point at which professional practice is indistinguishable from the state; part and parcel of governmentality.

LARSON AND FOUCAULT: EXPERTISE AND GOVERNMENTALITY

In order to extricate ourselves from the distorting consequences of the state/profession dualism, we must first rid our thinking of the concept of the state as a preconstituted, calculating subject. We must also develop a more balanced view of both the state and the professions as the structured outcomes of political objectives and governmental programmes rather than seeing them as either the constraining environments of action or the preconstituted agents of action. We can move further in this direction by considering the significance for our argument of the work of sociologists Larson (1977) and Abbott (1988), both of whom emphasize the processual nature of the social construction of expertise. Like Freidson, Larson and Abbott offer relatively sophisticated analyses of the professions, the former viewing professionalization as primarily the construction of a market in professional commodities or services; the latter identifying professionalism as a system of competitive occupational relations centring on jurisdictional claims and disputes.

For Larson, the market in professional services, as it emerged in the nineteenth century, depended on the production of a distinctive commodity. It being in the nature of a professional commodity to be inextricably 'bound to the person and personality of the producer' (Larson 1977: 14), it follows that the creation of a distinctive service requires the prior training, socialization and public establishment of a recognizable producer. Here, like Foucault, Larson links the emergence of the techniques and procedures of expertise to the reproduction of trained subjects. However, Foucault's analysis takes a different course to that of Larson, focusing on the normalization of the self-regulating, subject-client (the client, patient), rather than the subject-producer (the expert, professional). Foucault is interested in the general process of governmentality; its disciplines and its objects. Larson is concerned with the construction and institutionalization of expertise; one strand of governmentality.

For Larson the creation of an established market in professional commodities required that 'stabled criteria of evaluation' were fixed in the minds of consumer-clients. This process of commodity standardization was associated with the elimination of alternative criteria of evaluation and, therefore, of alternative practitioners. Larson, in keeping with other sociologists, regards the elimination of 'quacks' as centrally significant to the monopolization of expertise associated with professionalization. But Foucault once again shifts our attention to the governing process and its dependence on the establishment of uniform definitions of reality. Larson, by stressing the professional drive towards practice monopoly, tends to underplay the importance for the governing process of the establishment of universally recognized definitions of social reality. As Miller and Rose point out, such definitions render

> aspects of existence thinkable and calculable, and amenable to deliberate and planful initiatives; a complex intellectual labour involving not only the invention of new forms of thought, but also the invention of novel procedures of documentation, computation and evaluation.

> (1990: 3)

It is in such a context that the existence of competing forms of expertise not only undermines the professionalizing strategies of occupations, but also reduces the coherence of government programmes.

Larson (1977: 14–18) comes close to Foucault when she suggests that in the development of the modern professions commodity standardization was but one aspect of a wider process of 'ideological persuasion', itself part of a newly emerging symbolic universe. According to Larson (1977: 15), the state, 'the supreme legitimising and enforcing institution', was fundamental to securing the conditions of professionalization. The 'conquest of official privilege' was essential in constructing that public 'monopoly of credibility' (Larson 1977: 17) which today remains central to the creation of a professional commodity. However favoured an occupation might be in the division of labour, the creation of a realm of cognitive exclusiveness as part of a successful project of market control depended on the supporting role of the state. Larson quotes Polyani (1957) approvingly:

> the road to the free market was opened and kept open by an enormous increase in continuous, centrally organized and controlled interventionism. . . . There was nothing natural about laissez-faire . . . laissez-faire itself was enforced by the state.
>
> (1977: 53)

State-backed monopoly was, Larson claims, the mechanism through which professions 'protected themselves against the undue interference of the state' (1977: 53).

In seeking to explain the rise of the professions, then, Larson comes to much the same conclusion as Freidson; that it is state intervention or 'shelter' that secures professional autonomy – the paradox is restated. As with Freidson, the value of Larson's analysis lies in the fact that she also refuses to sit secure on one or other side of the dualist see-saw of state intervention and professional autonomy. In Larson's analysis autonomy depends on intervention, not on this occasion because autonomy and intervention refer to two different objects (that is, technical evaluation as against socio-economic organization) but because intervention is construed as a class strategy in which state intervention favours the bourgeoisie – in this case the professional segment of the bourgeoisie: 'Indeed, reliance upon the state was not merely a pattern borrowed by the nineteenth-century professions from the medieval guilds, but also the means by which the ascending bourgeoisie had advanced toward a self-regulating market' (Larson 1977: 53). There is in Larson's account, then, no necessity for autonomy to be built into the technicality of expertise. Rather, professional autonomy is seen as an historical emergent; part of the processes of class and state formation. By stressing the historical specificity of professionalization and its links to state and class formation Larson draws a little closer to Foucauldian analysis. However, her argument is of particular value when she introduces Gramscian theory to suggest that: 'Intellectuals are obviously of strategic importance for the ruling class, whose power cannot rest on coercion alone but needs to capture the moral and intellectual direction of society as a whole.' (Larson 1977: xiv).

This 'organic' tie to a rising class identifies professionals as potentially privileged bodies of experts, officially entrusted with the task of defining a sector of reality in a way that underpins established or emergent power; whether that be conceived of as state power or class power. This reference to Gramsci identifies an important aspect of the profession/state complex that is often noted, but only emerges as a systematic concern in Foucauldian analysis. Namely, the fact that expertise not only functions as a system of legitimation, but is institutionalized as part of the governing and legitimating processes.

While both Larson and Freidson emphasize that professional expertise has been dependent on governments for recognition, licence and legitimation, they are not so systematically emphatic that the professions, in constructing an officially recognized realm of social reality, are also a significant source of the growing capacity for governing, expressed by Foucault in the concept of governmentality. Foucault's argument deepens our understanding of these inter-dependencies of class, state and professions, by focusing on what Larson refers to as the 'new symbolic universe' associated with the rise of the professions. This emergent pattern of cognitive and normative changes – the 'great transformation' – not only generated the popular legitimations underpinning liberal, democratic government, but also induced what Stanley Cohen (1985), after Foucault, has called a profound shift in the 'master patterns of social control'. This shift included the construction of new deviancy control systems, the institutional expressions of which were the 'austere' and 'rational' bureaucratic organizations created for the classification and segregation of the poor, the criminal, the mad, the sick and the young. It is from Foucault that we derive the view that government and the professions were inextricably fused in this 'transformation' of the 'strategies and technologies' of power. Both were the progenitors and, in part, the beneficiaries of this complex network of interrelated social realities which constituted the various emergent realms of expertise and rendered them governable.

If at this stage of the argument we continue to insist on the dualism, state/profession, the word juggling becomes extreme. For we are forced to conclude not only that the independence of the professions depends on the interventions of the state, but that the state is dependent on the independence of the professions in securing the capacity to govern as well as legitimating its governance. The obvious implication of all this is to suggest that we must develop ways of talking about state and profession that conceive of the relationship not as a struggle for autonomy or control but as the interplay of integrally related structures, evolving as the combined product of occupational strategies, governmental policies and shifts in public opinion.

ABBOTT AND FOUCAULT: REALMS OF EXPERTISE AND GOVERNMENTALITY

This conclusion brings us to Abbott's *The System of Professions*, a recent and fruitful sociological perspective, worth considering here insofar as it insists that the 'real, the determining history of the professions' (1988: 2) lies in competitive struggles between occupations for jurisdiction over realms of expertise. Accord-ing to Abbott, experts are continuously engaged in making claims and counter-claims for jurisdiction over existing, emergent and vacant areas of expertise. These are the very same realms of expertise that Foucault identifies as enabling and empowering governmentality. In short, far from avoiding politics by way of the adoption of a neutral stance or the establishment of autonomy, professionals are always, in their jurisdictional competitions, intimately involved in politics; the politics of governmentality.

The value of Abbott's approach for us lies not so much in his focus on the professions as a 'system' of such competitive relationships, but in the claim that the established professions – institutionalized expertise – are emergent from such a competitive, political process. Abbott advances beyond the conventional socio-logical literature, then, in focusing *not* on the preconstituted professional subject seeking autonomy, but on the processes through which occupations constitute and reproduce themselves, relative to others, as professions.

The degree to which this approach, by focusing on the political process of jurisdictional claims, suggests a dismemberment of the intervention/autonomy couple is once again undermined by Abbott's insistence on the duality of state and profession. For example, Abbott's model suggests that the system of compe-titive interdependencies that generates a profession has its origins in negotiated jurisdictions in the workplace; jurisdictions which are thereafter generalized through the establishment of such claims first in the arena of public opinion and then in the legal order (Abbott 1988: 59–61); this last linking nicely with the problematic of governmentality. In Abbott's analysis, however, it is only at the point at which the legal order is brought into play that the state emerges, as a preconstituted, calculating subject.

The state is conceived largely as an audience for professional claims. In other words the state is an environmental factor in the system of professions; an external agent made up of the legislature, the courts and the administrative or planning structure (Abbott 1988: 62–3). The typical sequence of events in the establishment of a professional jurisdiction involves the success of an occupation in workplace negotiations, followed by an accepted claim in the public arena of opinion, and only then a 'crowning' of these earlier successes by way of legal recognition.

The initial problem that arises for such an analysis is that it is difficult to sustain the validity of this sequence of events for the development of the pro-fessions in any country other than the United States. However, according to Abbott, while the sequence is crucial in establishing professional claims in the United States, in a number of continental European countries the state rather than public opinion has, untypically, constituted the primary audience for juris-dictional claims. In these cases, he argues, public opinion coalesces with the administration and the legal order to constitute the 'common opinion of state officials' (Abbott 1988: 60).

By identifying the state in terms of its organizational locations (the courts, legislature, administration) and its interventionist capacity (Abbott 1988: 163), and by separating both of these from the arena of public opinion, Abbott leaves himself with no effective means of incorporating the wider politics of state formation into his jurisdictional analysis, despite the fact that his work leads one in that very direction. In short, the reactive state (pro-active in the case of France (Abbott 1988: 158–62) is divorced from the public arena, while work-site negotiations are cut off from public and national processes of claim and counter-claim. Abbott's concept of 'audiences' for professional claims cuts across the field of political struggles, so submerging their effects.

For Foucault the concept of governmentality incorporates the politics of expertise, which are, at one and the same time, made up of Abbott's occupational competition over jurisdictions, the politics of policy formation and the politics of state formation. If we recognize that both public opinion and government con-stitute, along with the experts themselves, agents in a political process, then we must reject the implication in Abbott's analysis that governments are typically latecomers on the scene, uninvolved in the formation of public opinion or the work-site formation of occupational jurisdictions.

In centring his analysis on the interplay of jurisdictional claims, Abbott focuses on the professions as an emergent set of properties arising out of occupational strategies. The state remains conceptualized as a preconstituted, reactive agent rather than itself an emergent property of the system. Once we include governments and administrators as participating equally with the experts in Abbott's complex of jurisdictional claims, then we also describe part of the process that Foucault calls governmentality. Once we follow Foucault in concep-tualizing the state as the outcome of these interrelations, then we can begin to look at the issues associated with the institutionalization of expertise in a manner quite other than that imposed on us by the state intervention/professional auto-nomy couple.

One result of such a reconceptualization will be the recognition that the 'neutrality' of professional expertise, where it exists, is itself an outcome of a political process rather than the product of some inherent essence, such as esoteric knowledge. Once we see institutionalized expertise as an aspect of governmentality then it is possible to recognize that professionalization begins not only with the adoption of occupational strategies, but also with the formation of government programmes and objectives.

STARR AND IMMERGUT: THE CHANGING BOUNDARIES OF POLITICS

These issues can be elaborated further by way of a consideration of yet another recent contribution to the sociology of the professions, the article by Starr and Immergut (1987) on 'Health care and the boundaries of politics'. Their thesis, relating to governmental health policies, effectively resituates Abbott's argument regarding the establishment of professional jurisdictions by focusing on politics as a sphere in which various interests, groups and individuals struggle over and 'seek to shape the uses of governmental power' (Starr and Immergut 1987: 222). This contribution brings us closer to the Foucauldian perspective insofar as governmentality is an attempt to specify the nature of government power in modern societies.

According to Starr and Immergut the general sphere of politics has the capacity to expand and contract. In periods of rapid social change, for example, arenas of decision-making once considered realms of neutral, objective fact may be reconstituted as politically contentious. That is to say, matters which Freidson might identify as of purely technical concern – to be resolved by recognized experts – erupt into 'political controversy'.

In Britain, we have recently experienced a number of such eruptions, largely as a result of the Thatcher government's policy initiatives of the 1980s; policies affecting a variety of professions including medicine, education, law and planning. As long ago as 1974 Sir Keith Joseph, the first Thatcherite Minister of Education, indicated what was to come when he made the following comments on planning and planners:

> It is not only that the pursuit of town planning aims intensifies land shortage, prolongs delays, increases devastation, imposes rigid lifeless solutions; it is not only that town planning makes the artificial shortages that lead to the fortunes that feed envy; it is not only that the ambitious system of town planning leads to long administrative delays with heavy concealed costs all round on top of the visible costs of a big bureaucracy; it is not only that any system leading to such wide disparities of land values must offer a temptation to corruption; it is that town planners and architects are as fallible as the rest of us and the more power we give them the greater errors that will be made when they are wrong.
>
> (quoted in Cherry 1982: 69)

Joseph's attack represented a rupture of the postwar political consensus which viewed professional town planning as one of the glories of the welfare state. His remarks also drew on an immense well of public disillusionment over urban town planning in particular (Dennis 1972), and a growing scepticism about the role of the professions in general.

The implications of Joseph's remarks did not emerge fully, however, until the third term of the Thatcher government, when the elements that made up the overall policy towards expert services began to fall into place – the Education Reform Bill, the Health Services White Paper, the Green Paper on Legal Services, the White Paper on the Reorganization of Broadcasting, and the Monopoly and Mergers Commission Reports on professional advertising. Together these events constituted an unprecedented shake-up in the jurisdictions and organization of expert services, with potential effects rivalling the privatizations of state-run industries.

The overall objectives of government policy also became increasingly clear. While the government was attempting to achieve a variety of specific policy goals relating to the provision of legal services, the stock market, the National Health Service, the universities and the schools, each of these cases also illustrated an overall policy commitment to cost effectiveness, accountability, competition and consumer choice. The common assumption behind each discrete reform was that the high and spiralling costs of expert services – some argued of professional privilege – were no longer acceptable.

A rapidly ageing population rendered the problem of cost particularly acute in the field of health care. The legal services were increasingly threatened by the pressure on legal aid, while in further and higher education the government's commitment to a policy of rapid expansion threatened a further cost explosion. The government's response to these compounded issues was the establishment of systems of monitoring, audit and appraisal as means of controlling costs. Whether applied by the professionals themselves or by external agencies these systems have, along with associated policies, the potential to redefine the boundaries between professional occupations, as well as the relations between professionals and their clients. In many cases it is too early to assess the full effects of such reforms, but it is clear that the boundaries defining expert jurisdictions and realms of neutrality are in process of transformation.

For example, the systems of financial and medical audit developed in respect of general practice and hospitals in the National Health Service have become hot political issues, centred on the competing criteria of 'cost' and 'care'. Cost criteria, it has been argued by the medical profession, are likely to distort the clinical judgements of general practitioner budget-holders, particularly in respect of the elderly and the chronically ill, who would become a drain on practice budgets funded in accordance with an undifferentiated per capita rate. What were once accepted as technical matters best determined within the confines of the general practitioner's consulting room have become burning political issues. The point is that changing government objectives have had the effect of shifting the boundaries between what was regarded as contentious and what was accepted as neutral. To put it in another way, the arenas of professional neutrality and autonomy are transformed, not as a product of changing occupational strategies, as Abbott would have it; not as an effect of technical change, as suggested by Freidson; but as a result of changing government objectives and policies.

As government objectives alter, transforming the boundaries of politics, so too do professional jurisdictions and the established powers and functions of the state. The point is central to Foucault's view of governmentality:

> [Since] it is the tactics of the government which make possible the continual definition and redefinition of what is within the competence of the State and what is not, the public versus the private, and so on; thus the State can only be understood in its survival and its limits on the basis of the general tactics of governmentality.
>
> (Foucault 1979: 21)

The processes as described by Starr and Immergut are just these tactics of governmentality. They are the policy-triggered politicizations and depoliticizations which constantly 'disturb established rights and powers' (Starr and Immergut 1987: 222), including those of experts. A crucial aspect of what they call the 'permanent structure' of the modern liberal state are the boundaries which conventionally and legally demarcate distinctions between the public and the private, between the technical and the political and, it follows, between the professions and the state:

> [Professional] or administrative sphere in government, which they hold separate from politics. Indeed, the military, civil service, scientific agencies and public health services are generally not only thought but legally required to be divorced from politics in the restricted but important sense of being nonpartisan and professional.
>
> (Starr and Immergut 1987: 225)

The authors make it clear that the notion of boundary is, in their usage, merely a spatial metaphor which lends 'an exaggerated fixity' to these distinctions which are in reality 'ambiguous, multiple and overlapping' (Starr and Immergut, 1987: 251) as well as being politically and intellectually contested. Nevertheless, it remains the case that in modern democracies such boundaries are maintained even when, as observation shows, they are characterized by continuous movement. In short, those outcomes of governmentality we call the state, including those bodies of experts and expertise that both make it up yet are differentiated from it, are always in process of *becoming*.

EXPERTISE AND THE STATE

This is an important conclusion, for not merely does it suggest that we have commonly and mistakenly reified the state, but in so doing we have placed at the centre of our analyses concepts which misunderstand the nature of the empirical world. That is to say, we cannot understand what is happening to the professions today if we frame our questions around the issues of autonomy and intervention. Foucault redirects our attention to the place of expertise in the politics of governmentality: to the recognition of changing spheres of neutrality and technicality, as identified by Starr and Immergut; to the generation of novel disciplines that both define and render governable realms of social reality, as underscored by Larson; to the establishment of these disciplines as part of a process of struggle over jurisdictional claims and occupational strategies, as outlined by Abbott.

If we also take from Starr and Immergut the notion that definitions of the technical and the political – that is, their boundaries – are constantly in process of transformation, then it follows that Freidson's view that the distinctive feature of a profession, autonomy in controlling its own technical work, is always contingent. This does not damage Freidson irretrievably for, as Larson points out, the implication of much of his analysis is that the cognitive and normative elements so crucial to the defining of a profession 'should not be viewed as stable and fixed characteristics' (Larson 1977: xii). What is important here, however, is that the illegitimacy of 'external evaluation' must also be understood not as an established universal but as an historical emergent requiring constant reinforcement, renegotiation and re-establishment within the context of changing government programmes. Autonomy as an outcome of political processes, far from being reduced by 'state intervention', is a product of governmentality that brings the state into being. In short, Freidson's position can be sustained only when we rid him of the concept of the state as an interventionist subject.

The Foucauldian perspective also suggests that those cognitive and normative elements which Freidson and others see statically, as establishing the boundaries between associations of professional experts and the state, must be viewed processually as means or weapons in the struggle to define the boundaries of the technical and political; the means of negotiation used by politicians and officials as well as professionals in generating those discourses that define the possible realms of governance. Professional men and women have, for example, routinely mobilized their claims to expertise and technicality as means of establishing and sustaining an arena of independent action. The doctors use their claim to diagnostic inviolability as a weapon in the effort to influence government policy. The outcome of the battle between the Royal Colleges and the British Medical Association, on the one hand, and the British government, on the other, over the reform of the National Health Service is just one phase in this continuous political process determining not only the future of that service but also the future lineaments of medical expertise and the future powers and capacities of the state.

Since the emergence of modern, liberal-democratic government expertise has become a key resource of 'governmentality'; that is, the technical and institutional capacity to exercise a highly complex form of power. Governmentality has been associated with the official recognition and licence of professional expertise as part of a general process of implementing government objectives and standardizing procedures, programmes and judgements. Also, because governments depend on the neutrality of expertise in rendering social realities governable, the established professions have been, as far as possible, distanced from spheres of political contention – the source of professional autonomy. However, because government policies and policy objectives change over time, these boundaries are in constant flux, having the effect of refashioning jurisdictions, breaking down arenas and neutrality and constructing new ensembles of procedures, techniques, calculations and roles which reconstitute the lineaments of the state itself.

The Thatcherite reforms in Britain, while changing the relationships between professions as they have between such groups as solicitors and barristers, solicitors and estate agents, and bankers and solicitors, are likely in the longer term to bring new jurisdictional claimants into being. Among the potential claimants are the ranks of appraisers, auditors and monitors of expert services. The current efforts to construct the discipline of appraisal not only opens up new jurisdictions relating to such expertise, it also opens up the potential for a re-articulation of the relations between all experts and the state in ways which might well corrode the existing conditions of occupational autonomy or even undermine professionalism as the characteristic institutional form. Once we recognize the symbiotic form of professionalization and state formation it also becomes clear that any modern government that pursues policies with the effect of politicizing established areas of expertise and destabilizing existing professional jurisdictions also risks undermining the entrenched conditions that sustain legitimate official action. For example, the universities, while often providing a social space for the expression of dissent, have also in the modern era been an increasingly significant source of expert authority in support of government programmes. They have been particularly significant in securing the conditions of governmentality by providing an independent system of certification. The university degree is accepted as a valid measure of individual, cognitive variation; part of the process of normalization that renders inequality entirely 'natural'; a reflection of inner merit. A potential source of social dissension is deflected out of the political sphere. When governments undermine the neutrality of such processes they also tamper with the conditions required by governmentality.

The concept of the state that emerges from this discussion includes, then, that multiplicity of regulatory mechanisms and instrumentalities that give effect to government. This state itself emerges out of a complex interplay of political activities, including the struggle for occupational jurisdictions. The state forms, in the context of the exercise of power, systems of technique and instrumentality: of notation, documentation, evaluation, monitoring and calculation, all of which function to construct the social world as arenas of action. It is in the context of such processes that expertise in the form of professionalism becomes part of the state. Expert technologies, the practical activities of professional occupations, and the social authority attaching to professionalism are all implicated in the process of rendering the complexities of modern social and economic life knowable, practicable and amenable to governing.

The professions, then, are involved in the constitution of the objects of politics; in the identification of new social problems, the construction of the means or instrumentalities for solving them, as well as in staffing the organizations created to cope with them. The professions become, in this view, socio-technical devices through which the means and even the ends of government are articulated. In rendering a realm of affairs *governable*, whether it be education, law, health or even in shaping the self-regulating capacity of subjectivity among citizens, the professions are a key resource of governing in a liberal-democratic state.

REFERENCES

Abbott, A. (1988) *The System of Professions: An Essay on the Division of Expert Labor*, Chicago: University of Chicago Press.

Barber, B. (1963) 'Some problems in the sociology of the professions', *Daedalus* Fall: 669–88.

Bell, D. (1960) *The End of Ideology*, Glencoe, Ill.: Free Press.

Cherry, G. (1982) *The Politics of Town Planning*, London: Longman.

Cohen, S. (1985) *Visions of Social Control*, Cambridge: Polity Press.

Dennis, N. (1972) *Public Participation and Planners' Blight*, London: Faber.

Derber, C. (ed.) (1982) *Professionals as Workers: Mental Labor in Advanced Capitalism*, Boston: G. K. Hall.

Foucault, M. (1973) *Madness and Civilization: A History of Insanity in the Age of Reason*, London: Random House.

—— (1979) 'On governmentality', *Ideology and Consciousness* 6: 5–22.

Freidson, E. (1970) *Profession of Medicine: A Study in the Sociology of Applied Knowledge*, New York: Dodd, Mead & Co.

—— (1973) 'Professionalization and the organization of middle-class labour in post-industrial society', in P. Halmos (ed.), *Professionalization and Social Change*, Sociological Review Monograph No. 20: 47–60.

Haug, M. (1973) 'Deprofessionalization: an alternative hypothesis for the future', in P. Halmos (ed.), *Professionalization and Social Change*, Sociological Review Monograph No. 20: 195–212.

Larson, M. S. (1977) *The Rise of Professionalism: A Sociological Analysis*, Berkeley: University of California Press.

Lewis, R. and Maude, A. (1952) *Professional People*, London: Phoenix House.

Light, D. W. and Levine, S. (1988) 'The changing character of the medical profession: a theoretical overview', *The Milbank Quarterly* 66 (Suppl. 2): 10–32.

McKinlay, J. B. and Stoeckle, J. D. (1988) 'Corporatization and the social transformation of doctoring', *International Journal of Health Services* 18(2): 191–205.

Miller, P. and Rose, N. (1990) 'Governing economic life', *Economy and Society* 19(1): 1–31.

Navarro, V. (1976) *Medicine under Capitalism*, New York: PRODIST.

Oppenheimer, M. (1973), 'The proletarianization of the professional', in P. Halmos (ed.), *Professionalization and Social Change*, Sociological Review Monograph No. 20: 213–38.

Parsons, T. (1949), 'The professions in the social structure', in T. Parsons *Essays in Sociological Theory*, Glencoe, Ill.: Free Press.

Polanyi, K. (1957) *The Great Transformation*, Boston: Beacon Press.

Scull, A. T. (1979) *Museums of Madness*, London: Penguin Books.

Starr, P. and Immergut, E. (1987) 'Health care and the boundaries of politics', in C. S. Maier (ed.), *Changing Boundaries of the Political*, Cambridge: Cambridge University Press.

Wright, E. O. (1978) *Class, Crisis and the State*, London: New Left Books.

2 Countervailing powers

A framework for professions in transition

Donald Light

The professions today are experiencing one of their most turbulent periods, not only because of changes due to the internal dynamics of elaboration and segmentation, but also because markets, corporations and the state are undergoing profound transitions. This chapter presents a new concept and method for thinking about and analysing these changes. It builds on previous work which shall be referenced for the interested reader as the concept unfolds. Yet much further research and analysis is needed to develop the concepts and to test hypotheses derived from them.

Prevailing concepts of the professions, especially in regard to medicine, suffer from characterizing the sociological nature of the profession in terms of a certain endpoint or trend at a certain time in history. 'Professional dominance', 'proletarianization' and 'deprofessionalization' are examples of this problem. When viewed historically, prevailing concepts of a period are products of their time presented as timeless verities (Light 1989). As a result, these concepts do not frame the historical dynamics between professions and the state or governments. Light and Levine (1988), for example, analysed the ways in which the concepts of professional dominance, deprofessionalization, proletarianization, and its de-Marxed cousin, corporatization, each capture some aspects of professions today but characterize one tendency or trend for the entire dynamic relationship between profession and society. Each of these four characterizations is also relatively static and leaves little room for a sense of historical irony about the ways in which unanticipated consequences result from them. Of particular importance are the ironic consequences of professional dominance, as a profession's power to shape its domain in its own image leads to excesses that prompt counter-reactions (Light 1991a, 1991b, 1994).

THE CONCEPT AND ITS ORIGINS

The concept of countervailing powers first came to mind from analysing the development of the German health care system and the evolving shifts of power between profession and state from the l880s to the l980s (Light *et al.* 1986; Light and Schuller 1986; Light 1994). The sickness funds, having won the right to administer Bismarck's health insurance plan, became so dominant in their control of medical work that they prompted militant counter-reactions by private practitioners. Through hundreds of boycotts and strikes, they wrested many concessions and powers. Still dissatisfied, they continued to seek full control of medical services but did not succeed until they provided extensive support for Adolf Hitler, who neutralized the sickness funds in terms of organizational power and finally granted doctors the legal status of a profession under German law. There are probably few other cases where a profession has risen so completely from being the weakest party to the strongest in the field of organizational, political and economic forces that make up a professional domain. Militancy and dictatorial state support certainly helped.

Professional dominance, however, has produced its own excesses during the post-Second World War period: increasing specialization, elaboration of techniques and technology, spiralling costs, and the neglect of prevention and chronic care. As a result, the sickness funds and the West German state began to take counter-measures in the late 1970s to redress the imbalances. These have become increasingly structural and fundamental, culminating (so far) in the sweeping changes of 1993 (Light 1994). The dynamic relations between profession and state will, of course, continue to unfold.

This study proposes the concept of countervailing powers as a conceptual framework that allows us to organize and understand profession–state relations, but in such a way as to allow changes to be traced over time. Montesquieu (1748) first developed the idea of countervailing powers in his treatise about the abuses of absolute power by the state and the need for counterbalancing centres of power. Sir James Steuart (1767) contributed ironic observations of how the monarch's promotion of commerce to enhance its domain and wealth produced the countervailing power of the mercantile class that tempered the absolute power of the monarchy and produced a set of interdependent relationships. One might discern a certain analogy to the way in which the medical profession encouraged the development of pharmaceutical and medical technology companies to enhance professional powers in the markets of medicine. These corporations have enhanced the profession and extended its domain, but increasingly on their terms so that the profession serves their goals of growth and profit.

The broader sociological concept of countervailing powers builds on the work of Johnson (1972) and Larson (1977), who analysed distinct relations between profession, state and market in particularly suggestive ways. It focuses attention on the *interactions* of powerful actors in a field where they are inherently interdependent yet distinct. If one party is dominant, as the American medical profession has long been, its dominance is contextual and eventually elicits counter-moves by other powerful actors, not to destroy it but to redress an imbalance of power. '[P]ower on one side of a market', wrote John Kenneth Galbraith (1956: 113) in his original treatise on the dynamics of countervailing power in oligopolistic markets, 'creates both the need for, and the prospect of reward to the exercise of countervailing power from the other side'. In those states where the government has played a central role in nurturing professions within the state structure but has allowed the professions to establish their own institutions and power base, the professions and the state go through phases of harmony and discord in which countervailing actions take place. In states where the medical profession has been largely suppressed, we now see their rapid reconstitution once governmental oppression is lifted.

The time frame for countervailing moves is years or decades when political and institutional powers are involved. Dominance slowly produces imbalances, excesses and neglects that anger other countervailing (latent) powers and alienate the larger public. These imbalances include (1) internal elaboration and expansion that weaken the dominant institution from within; (2) a subsequent tendency to consume more and more of the nation's wealth; (3) a self-regarding importance that ignores the concerns of clients and institutional partners; and (4) an expansion of control that exacerbates the impact of the other three. Other characteristics of a profession which affect its relations with countervailing powers include (5) the degree and nature of competition with adjacent professions, about which Andrew Abbott (1988) has written with such richness; (6) the changing technological base of its expertise; and (7) the demographic composition of its membership.

As a sociological concept, countervailing powers is not confined to buyers and sellers but includes major political, social and other economic groups which contend with each other for legitimacy, prestige and power as well as for markets and money. Deborah Stone (1988) and Theodore Marmor and Jonathan Christianson (1982) have written insightfully about the ways in which countervailing powers attempt to portray benefits to themselves as benefits for everyone, or to portray themselves as the unfair and damaged victims of other powers (particularly the state), or to keep issues out of public view. Here, the degree of power consists of one's ability to override, suppress or render as irrelevant the challenges by others, either behind closed doors or in public.

Because the sociological concept of countervailing powers recognizes several parties and not just buyers and sellers, it opens the door to alliances between two or more parties. These alliances, however, are often characterized by *structural ambiguities*, a term based on Merton and Barber's (1976) concept of sociological ambivalence that refers to the cross-cutting pressures and expectations experienced by an institution in its relations to other institutions. For example, a profession's relationships to the corporations that supply it with equipment, materials and information technology both benefit the profession and make it dependent in uneasy ways. The corporations can even come to control professional practices in the name of 'quality'. Alliances with dominant political parties (Krause 1988; Jones 1991) or with governments are even more fraught with danger. The alliance of the German medical profession with the National Socialist Party, for example, though important to establishing its legitimacy, led to a high degree of governmental control over its work and even its professional knowledge base (Jarausch 1990; Light *et al.* 1986).

A MODEL OF COUNTERVAILING POWERS

A graphic model of countervailing powers might begin with a horizontal axis, with professional dominance on one end and state dominance on the other, crossed by a vertical axis with independently employed professionals at one end and state employed professionals at the other as in Figure 2.1. This follows the lead of Larkin (1988: 128), that state involvement need not preclude professional dominance and that relations between state and profession involved 'countervailing pressures'. The following paragraphs develop the indicated end points of the horizontal and vertical axes.

Professional dominance, in Freidson's original formulation (1970a, 1970b), meant not just control over professional work but also the use of this core control to attain dominance over finance, institutional structures, related powers and privileges, cultural charisma, and even the reconstruction of social realities as various crimes and sins became reconceptualized as illnesses. One can play out the implications: high status, high income, control over recruitment, training, certification, jobs, careers, facilities, equipment, and of course the organization of work. An important part of professional dominance is the elaboration of professional work, the power and resources (and mandate) to develop it to its highest, most sophisticated forms.

State dominance at the right end of the axis in Figure 2.1 stands for a situation perhaps like that in the former Soviet Union, where doctors are employees – with relatively low status and pay – of a delivery system designed by the state (Field 1988, 1991). They have little budgetary control and the budget is small, thus limiting professional elaboration, which is so critical to institutional elaboration and charismatic development. The state controls supply, most of the resources, and even the division of labour. The professionals in high office are political appointments whose job is to carry out the interest of the state, not the profession. The organized profession in this extreme, ideal-typical case is outlawed (Light, Leibfried and Tennstedt 1986).

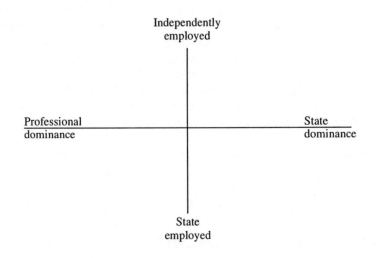

Figure 2.1 A profession's relations with the state

The right end of the axis need not be 'the state'. It can be an institution like the army, or a corporation like the United States lumber and railroad companies of the nineteenth century that employed large numbers of doctors to work in a medical service they totally controlled. Company doctors are coming back in the United States, in much more sophisticated and respectable forms (Walsh 1987). The right end of the axis can also be a payer like a sickness fund or insurance company or employer, or in one case a political party (Krause 1988). They can either hire doctors, put them on a retainer or pay them by procedure. One may therefore need several overlaying figures to analyse the locus and changing positions within a single system between the profession and other institutions.

THE NATURE OF AUTONOMY AND CONTROL

Setting up the horizontal axis of Figure 2.1 challenges a theoretical point made by Freidson (1970a: 25) long ago and sustained ever since. He stated that so long as a profession controls (or has autonomy over) its own technical core of work, it is whole or autonomous, even though the state controls external resources like budgets and institutions. This theoretical distinction is not supported by the actual effects of external resources and powers on clinical work (Abbott 1988). Budgets and institutions deeply influence the character of the 'technical core' of professional work. For example, if state decisions mean that even community doctors lack basic medical supplies and drugs, as has been the case in Russia and elsewhere, then the clinical core of professional autonomy or control is deeply compromised. With no penicillin, the doctor cannot even stop an ordinary ear infection in a small child before it spreads to the brain. The mother rushes out of the office to seek someone who can, with the doctor standing helpless and humiliated at the door. Even in much milder cases where the payer restricts supply or access, the core professional work is affected either directly or in-directly. Conversely, a state that in effect gives the profession the powers to shape the delivery system, buy what it wants, order what services it wants, and be paid well for it greatly affects the nature of clinical work. Thus Freidson's attempts to distinguish technical autonomy from socio-economic dependency are naïve.

The symbiotic relationship between micro- and macro-controls over the terms of work takes us to a basic reframing of autonomy as the foundation for profes-sionals. Autonomy is a subset of control – control over one's own actions. Thus, the larger concept is control, and Figure 2.2 lays out the continuum of control. Autonomy is not the core concept in the theory of professions but the most self-anchored end of the control continuum. It became important because the state or other concerned parties could not judge the performance of the profes-sional at work (Light 1988). In this position, the state and patients had little choice but to grant autonomy in return for promises of quality and altruism and hope for the best. Autonomy, then, became a central attribute of professional-ization not because it was inherently so but because the external gaze could not penetrate professional work.

The implicit social contract between society or the state and a profession is that the profession *as a whole* will be granted autonomy, but that, like the guilds of old, it will monitor the quality of work of its members. In other words, collective autonomy implies control over the individual member's performance, and even the collective autonomy implies a desire to control frustrated by technological limitations. The problem, however, is that individual professionals then declare autonomy – short of lying, cheating, gross incompetence and criminal behaviour – from their professional bodies of oversight. They say, as guild members did not, 'I am a professional and therefore autonomous; so you have no right to monitor my work so long as I do not breach broad professional standards.'

With new techniques for evaluating clinical performance, however, the state or other institutional powers can know even more about the quality of work a professional does than the professional him/herself (Björkman 1989). External agents can now document his/her practice patterns over time and compare them with colleagues in the area or with standards set by the doctors' own specialty society or by specialty teams of clinical researchers. Medical informatics, clinical algorithms and the computer have not only penetrated professional work but also rationalized it. Thus theories of professionalism that rest on autonomy as their cornerstone need to be reconstructed from the ground up.

Figure 2.2 below also clarifies just what the concept 'professional dominance' means. Freidson (1989), in defending professional dominance as it has declined during the 1980s, shifted the emphasis of the term to mean dominance over just core professional work. Had the original work defined professional dominance in such a familiar and orthodox way, it would not itself have had such compelling power. Thus a dominant profession at the left end of Figure 2.1 controls not only its own work but also a range of related institutions, services, privileges and finances as indicated by the right end of Figure 2.2.

Another clarification concerns the relationship between type of dominance and type of employment. As the vertical axis of Figure 2.1 indicates, there is a correlation but not a necessary relationship. In many countries, the state has nurtured the professions in the royal court or seat of power, as experts who extend the ruler's governmentality. Terry Johnson ably makes this case in chapter 1. In terms of power and status, court or government professionals have often had higher status, higher pay, more resources and far more power than their 'independent' (actually more dependent) brethren practising in an office out in some town. As the latter hung out their name plate, made night calls and tried to get clients to pay their bills (a humiliating aspect of 'independence'), the state

Clinical autonomy	+	Fiscal autonomy	+	Practice autonomy	+	Organizational autonomy	+	Organizational control (dominance)	+	Institutional control (dominance)

Figure 2.2 Degrees of professional power and control

professionals attended the opening of this season's performance of *Figaro* and the champagne party that followed. Moreover, state professionals need not be minions. They may (or may not) have many of the powers of professional dominance.

These points need emphasizing because so much of the sociological literature in English has assumed the Anglo-American ideal of the autonomous independent professional as the theoretical centre for analysis, rather than as a cultural ideal by certain professions at certain times in history. This misconception has caused many to think that as doctors become more often employed, they are being made into proletarians or are becoming corporatized. They may, but they may not. We need to sustain greater critical distance.

MODELLING COUNTERVAILING POWERS

The implication of these observations is that all four corners of Figure 2.1 are conceivable, even likely to have occurred in one place or another. One could have independent professionals collecting fees in a state, corporate or institutional system that shapes their organization of work, and that pinches them through low fee schedules. Medicaid in the United States might be characterized this way. Certainly it belongs somewhere in the northeastern quadrant of Figure 2.1. One could have independent professionals who rule all they survey in the northwestern quadrant, as was the case for American doctors for many decades and to a considerable degree still is. One could have state- or institution-employed doctors in a state- or institution-dominated system, or in a system that they dominate from the inside, as already described. And, as is usually the case, one can have mixtures, such as the British National Health Service (NHS).

British general practitioners before 1990 might be placed at ten o'clock within the northwestern quadrant of Figure 2.3, fairly independent (though a national contract), and fairly dominant (though restricted by a tight budget). British consultants might be placed in the quadrant below half way out at eight o'clock as state employees, on fairly good lifetime salaries (with indexed pensions) and a considerable amount of control over their work and institutions, but still within a state framework that keeps resources very restricted. Some might place them at seven o'clock.

The larger point is that profession and state are in a symbiotic relationship, what Klein (1990) effectively depicts as 'the politics of the double bed'. A profession that carries out the work of a state system, like the NHS, means that both parties must 'find ways of accommodating the frustrations and resentments of both sides in the partnership, and to devise organizational strategies for containing conflicting interests' (Klein 1990: 700). As Klein observes, the state has the power to breach these accommodations when determined to weaken professionalism. Similar moments are occurring in Germany, the United States, Sweden, New Zealand and Japan. They represent a shift from protected professionalism to contracted professionalism, from autonomy and authority to accountability and performance, with managers in a pivotal middle position.

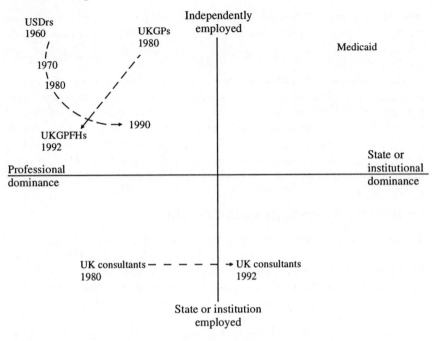

'USDrs' refers to office-based independent practitioners in the United States.
'UKGPs' refers to general practitioners in the United Kingdom.
'UKGPFHs' refers to general practitioner fundholders in 1992 in the United Kingdom. In the author's view, their increased dominance may be clipped in the next few years.
'UK consultants' refers to senior clinical specialists in the United Kingdom on a state salary.
'Medicaid' refers to independent doctors treating patients under the US programme for the poor.

Figure 2.3 Changing relations of British and American doctors with the state

The British transformation of its medical welfare system into contractual markets is shifting the positions of general practitioners and consultants (Light and May 1993). With fundholding, general practitioners are becoming more dominant but less independent, perhaps three-quarters of the way out at nine o'clock in Figure 2.3; and the consultants are getting weaker, perhaps moving towards five or six o'clock. In Germany, reforms have deepened from financial constraints and budgetary governance in the period from 1975 to the 1980s to restructuring the delivery system in the past five years and the next ten (Knox 1993; Light 1994). These structural changes are moving doctors rapidly from professional dominance at the left end of the horizontal axis of Figure 2.3 towards the centre. These brief examples illustrate the usefulness of the model, even though the exact placement can be debated.

EXPANDING THE MODEL TO MULTIPLE PARTIES

What makes the current era interesting is that the era of professional dominance in Western European countries and the United States, and of state dominance in Eastern European countries and the ex-Soviet Union, has come to an end. In most Western countries, professions have attained dominance, even inside state systems. The United States is the purest form of professional dominance, in which the entire legal and administrative structure reflects the priorities of the profession and provides protection for them. That is why the Americans have had such a difficult time controlling their costs since 1970, while the rest of the West has succeeded. As professional dominance developed its excesses, the United States had no state-level budgetary framework and the other countries did. As Freddi (1989: 12) puts it, the Europeans emphasize solidarity and equality, the Americans liberty and efficiency through market freedom. But aside from the exceptional case of the United States, professionalism has prevailed within the other Western health care systems. This is a point that Immergut (1992), in her elegant analytic study of political institutions and health policy, misses. Whether one looks at Sweden, with its strong executive state structure, or Switzerland, with its fragmented and veto-laced state structure, specialists and hospitals have captured most of the health care budget and prestige. The implicit ideal type of the profession is outlined in Table 2.1, a health care system aimed at providing the best clinical medicine to every sick patient and enhancing the stature of doctors. The priorities of this ideal type, their omissions as well as commissions, and their consequences for organization, power and finance have a good deal to do with the current efforts by states, employers, insurers and other payers to reduce professional dominance and harness professional work to their priorities. Wilsford has it right when he notes the transnational 'confrontation of scarce resources to pay health care with a rising demand for and technical capacity to provide care' (1991: 3).

What authors from Starr (1982) to Wilsford (1991) miss is the degree to which the era of professional dominance was (is) an imbalanced state among the countervailing powers in what W. Richard Scott (1993: 273) calls the 'organizational environment'. Dominance by either the profession or the state/institution 'bankrupts' the other major parties in various ways. This argument implies that the concept of countervailing powers is like the concept of conflict theory outlined by Coser (1954) in which the best state has only conflicts-in-equilibrium. The implication is that each party has legitimate goals and values which are not easy to fit with the others and which can lead to serious imbalances in their own right.

The medical profession wants to develop the best clinical medicine for every sick patient and enhance the stature of the profession. This meshes powerfully with what sick patients want except that the more they do, the more iatrogenic effects are likely. It does not mesh with what payers want, but payers also do not want to be seen as providing a skimpy or second-rate service to their citizens, employees or members. If professional dominance happens through the state, an

Table 2.1 The professional model of a health care system

Key values and goals	To provide the best possible clinical care to every sick patient (who can pay and who lives near where a doctor has chosen to practise). To develop scientific medicine to its highest level. To protect the autonomy of physicians and services. To increase the power and wealth of the profession. To increase the prestige of the profession.
Image of the individual	A private person who chooses how to live and when to use the medical system.
Power	Centres on the medical profession, and uses state powers to enhance its own.
Key institutions	Professional associations. Autonomous physicians and hospitals.
Organization	Centred on doctors' preferences of speciality, location and clinical cases. Emphasizes acute, hi-tech interventions. A loose federation of private practices and hospitals. Weak ties with other social institutions as peripheral to medicine.
Division of labour	Proportionately more doctors, more specialists. Proportionately more individual clinical work by physicians; less delegation.
Finance and costs	Private payments by individual or through passive reimbursement by insurance plans. Costs about twice the % GNP of the societal model. Doctors' share greater than societal model.
Medical education	Private, autonomous schools with tuition. Disparate, voluntary continuing education.

Note: 'Societal model' refers to another in the set found in Light (1994). It starts with the goal of maximizing health status and public health.

employer (company doctors) or now corporate payers in the United States, the medical élite gain great power at the expense of their rank-and-file subordinate colleagues; but that power is exercised in terms of the institution, be it Stalin or Hilter at the political extreme, or the principal stockholders of a for-profit corporation at the economic extreme. This situation results in great professional power and deprofessionalization simultaneously, what might be called *co-opted professional power*.

This analysis differs from that of Freidson (1989), who believes the profession as a whole is still dominant even though the rank and file increasingly must follow clinical protocols and guidelines, because doctors play central roles in developing those protocols and in running the delivery systems. This internal differentiation is certainly growing, but it does not contribute to maintaining dominance, because those doctors work for and develop the goals of the state or other major payer. To the extent that they are leaders of the profession, the profession as a whole gets corporatized through them, not the other way around. From the profession's point of view, not only practitioner autonomy but also the knowledge base, the character of work, and the organization of work are compromised, though this may be better overall for society. Analytically, this technical and managerial élite is similar to powerful political leaders recruiting a medical élite and giving them significant resources to advance their political ends, though emotionally the analogy is offensive.

If professional dominance happens on the profession's own terms, professionals regard it as ideal; but it too leads to distortions that eventually arouse other parties to redress the imbalances. Pursuing 'the best clinical medicine for every sick patient' leads to technical elaboration and specialization. The profession becomes organizationally embedded, and the organizational density of its practice increases (Freddi 1989: 4–12). These in turn drive up costs rapidly, make doctors dependent on those who can bankroll the large capitalization, require complex organizations which then spawn a new corps of professional managers, fragment political power, and inflate demand beyond what doctors can deliver, prompting law suits or other actions. Add to this a fierce insistence on independent practice, and a nation gets increased maldistribution by geography and specialty of services to needs. Great variations of practice arise, with no rational defence of more costly patterns.

The state or other institutional payers (such as employers and unions) constitute a second party. Their interests reflect Parsons' functional emphasis on keeping people functioning in their roles with as little costs and trouble as possible. (Insurers and benefits managers are agents of these parties.) Their principal concerns are governmentability and cost. However, state or payer dominance can be as imbalanced as professional dominance, leading to underfunding, depleting the profession of its capacity to do its job well, financial corruption, political corruption, depersonalized care and alienation (Jones 1991). The profession tries to limit the state's role to legitimation and sponsorship. State patronage enhances professional dominance; yet as Larkin (1988) points out, it can also curtail it. The end of professional dominance involves the state and other major payers entering the governance structure of the profession to monitor its work and restrain its economic and clinical activities (Freddi 1989: 25). The state's development of highly professional agencies that analyse health care practitioners more systematically than the practitioners themselves changes the balance of power fundamentally (Björkman 1989).

Patients as a third party also want to function in their roles, but, as Parsons suggested in his psychoanalytic model, they want some sympathy, indulgence, mothering or caring, and some rest to recover from illness or injury, even if it costs more. There is also a profoundly intense relation to one's body when it malfunctions or is assaulted that has origins too deep for sociology or medicine or even most psychology to comprehend. For many people in many cultures, any treatment at any cost is worthwhile if it promises recovery. This urgent need, however, can lead to the rise of quacks, charlatans and corrupted professionals as well as to great cost.

As the fourth party, the corporations that make up the medical-industrial complex want to maximize profits both short-term and long-term through constant product innovations and improvements, consumer fetishism (usually of doctors not patients), cornering markets, expanding current markets, creating new markets, large mark-ups, collusion and tying relations with doctors and medical centres that lock in business. (Many neo-classical economists seem to forget that the goal of competitors is to minimize competition by any means possible, that is, to undermine or distort the basic conditions for a good competitive market [Light 1990].)

These corporations seem to be the allies of the profession, and in all countries the medical profession has welcomed medical supply, pharmaceutical and medical equipment companies. Their innovations significantly enhance professional power regardless of how effective various procedures, machines, drugs and tests turn out to be. When they do not enhance the scientific base of medicine, they enhance its scientistic image. These allies, however, are exploiting the profession for high profits. The protected markets that professionalism creates are a capitalist's heaven. Moreover, health product corporations support many professional activities, from journals to continuing medical education, until the profession is deeply dependent on and corrupted by their interests. Several studies have shown that even though doctors believe their clinical decisions are not influenced by marketing, in fact they are. This is increasingly true of academic medicine, the centre of training and new knowledge on which so much of the profession rests. Figure 2.4 below depicts the corporate–state matrix in which academic medicine is enmeshed. Most professionals deny that their judgement has been compromised, but researchers find that it is. As for the state, the effects produce a profound ambivalence; for the economic success of the medical-industrial complex as it spurs doctors and patients to ever more elaborated medicine produces vigorous economic growth and mounting health care expenses.

These observations lead us from the simple scheme of professional vs state/institutional dominance in Figure 2.1 to the tetrahedron in Figure 2.5, in which each corner represents dominance by one of the four parties. The lines represent relative states of conflict and cooperation between pairs of parties, and the interior of the tetrahedron itself is the organizational field of countervailing powers (Scott 1993). If in other models there are more than four parties, such as nursing, chiropractic or acupuncture, then one needs a more complex polyhedron to depict it.

The concept of countervailing powers and these models will provide readers with a framework in which to place the chapters of this book on such topics as the changing power structure around general practice and community care, the impact of national policy in Spain, Britain and Eastern Europe, and changes in relations between health professions.

SOCIOLOGICAL MARKETS AND ECONOMIC COMPETITION

This conceptual development of countervailing powers provides a dynamic framework for understanding markets and their relations to a profession. The

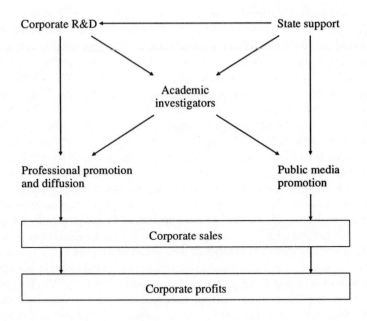

Figure 2.4 The state-academic-professional involvement in the medical-industrial complex

Source: Light (1993), based on Waitzkin (1983)

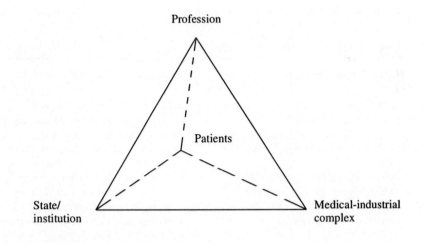

Figure 2.5 Multi-dimensional field of countervailing powers

market is the organizational field, the volume inside Figure 2.5. It is a socio-logical and political market as well as an economic one. Most authors and policy-makers today address a narrower subset, namely economic competition. Usually they mean an even narrower subset, monopsony competition fostered by the state or other major payers in order to break down the economic and institutional dominance of the profession (see Björkman 1989). The concept of 'the health care market' in Britain, the Netherlands, Sweden, Germany and elsewhere stems from neo-classical health economists (most notably Enthoven) promoting a special form of 'managed competition' as a tool or weapon for major payers to move the balance point along the horizontal axis of Figure 2.1, which is only one axis of Figure 2.5 (Glaser 1993). The three-dimensional space of Figure 2.5, however, allows us to depict the obvious, namely that the balance points are inside the figure and thus involve all four parties in interrelated ways. For example, to the extent that the state and/or other major payers restrict the budget for medical care (even if just to its current high level), it affects patients and the medical-industrial complex as well as the profession.

Market strategies as an economic tool by major payers fit poorly with profes-sional work for reasons long known and summarized in Table 2.2. The rhetoric about how the crisp, efficient and responsive discipline of markets will replace the clumsy, inefficient and unresponsive hierarchy of state bureaucracies is naïve. Economic competition usually allows providers to exploit the weaknesses listed in Table 2.2 and to drive costs up by pursuing their non-economic goals of providing the best clinical medicine to every sick patient.

In the more complex and esoteric aspects of work where the professions are usually found, however, economic markets work in very different but equally imperfect ways. So does the state. The 'products', their qualities and their costs are often difficult to define and measure. When they can be measured, they

Table 2.2 Perfect vs imperfect markets

Ideal of perfect markets	*Actual hazards of imperfect markets*
Transaction and market costs zero.	Large transaction and market costs.
Many buyers and sellers.	Few buyers and/or sellers. Market capture.
Nature, quality, effectiveness and price of products or service known. No market failure.	Nature, quality, effectiveness and/or price of products or service somewhat known and variable. Some market failure.
Power, rules, hiearchy, do not exist.	Power, rules, hierarchies found everywhere.
Manipulations, gaming, cost-shifting, unknown.	Manipulations, gaming, cost-shifting prevalent. Induced market failure.
Losers collapse, disappear.	Losers stay around. System carries their inefficiencies
Maximum efficiency.	Maximum inefficiencies?
Responsive to customers.	'Responsive' to customers. Induced demand, product or service dilution or substitution, misleading information.

usually are not, and comparative data by which buyers can shop for price, quality and features, like choosing a personal computer, are almost non-existent. Professional work is rife with competing 'schools of thought' which resolve by dint of personality and belief the many ambiguities of uncertainty about which method is the most effective (Light 1979). Ultimately, clients must depend on trust, on *confidat emptor* rather than *caveat emptor*. In these and many other ways, professional work fits poorly into an economic market model. The 'market' is sociological and political, involving norms, roles, power relations and hierarchy more than price. This analysis means that forms of what economists call 'market failure' are sociological patterns of interaction that only 'fail' in the sense of not fitting the narrow economic model. Thus, when Enthoven (1988) recognizes all the forms of 'market failure' in health care and then constructs managed competition as a way to get participants focused on price and efficiency, he is essentially contriving a system of rules to put hammerlocks on sociological patterns of behaviour by actors in health care so they will behave the way he wants them to.

These observations may imply that professionalism is a force in history and society not sufficiently recognized by neo-classical economists, by Marxists, or by theorists of the state. Although never wholly independent from the culture, political/legal structure and economy of a society, professions are a distinct, institutional power.

In economic theory, even in the more sociological explorations of Oliver Williamson which juxtapose markets and hierarchy in the search for efficiency, professionalism is not considered. Yet professionalism is a third option to markets and hierarchy, especially in complex situations enveloped in uncertainties. Professionalism uses dependency and trust in matters of complex skills and subtle judgement more efficiently than markets or hierarchy. The right product for a given problem is chosen and serviced by an expert more quickly and accurately than shopping in a market or having a hierarchy make a decision. 'Efficiency' is maximized, especially if one understands that most gains in so-called efficiency in health care come from increasing effectiveness. This point has been developed elsewhere (Cochrane 1972; Light 1991c).

To conclude, the predominantly sociological aspects of markets in health care are framed by the model of countervailing powers, providing a context in which to place what economists call market failure and their solutions to it. But a great deal more needs to be done to develop the legal, organizational and political dimensions to the countervailing powers model, and to develop empirical measures of its dynamics.

REFERENCES

Abbott, A. (1988) *The System of Professions: An Essay on the Division of Expert Labor*, Chicago: University of Chicago Press.
Björkman, J. W. (1989) 'Politicizing medicine and medicalizing politics: physician power in the United States', in G. Freddi and J. W. Björkman (eds), *Controlling Medical Professionals: The Comparative Politics of Health Governance*, London: Sage.

Cochrane, A. L. (1972) *Effectiveness and Efficiency*, London: Nuffield Provincial Hospitals Trust.

Coser, L. A. (1954) *The Functions of Social Conflict*, New York: Free Press.

Enthoven A. C. (1988) *Theory and Practice of Managed Competition in Health Care Finance*, Amsterdam: North-Holland.

Field, M. G. (1988) 'The position of the Soviet physician: the bureaucratic professional', *The Milbank Quarterly* 66 (Suppl. 2): 182–201.

Field, M. G. (1991) 'The hybrid profession: Soviet medicine', in A. Jones (ed.), *Professions and the State: Expertise and Autonomy in the Soviet Union and Eastern Europe*, Philadelphia: Temple University Press.

Freddi, G. (1989) 'Problems of organizational rationality in health systems: political controls and policy options', in G. Freddi and J. W. Björkman (eds), *Controlling Medical Professionals: The Comparative Politics of Health Governance*, London: Sage.

Freidson, E. (1970a) *Profession of Medicine: A Study in the Sociology of Applied Knowledge*, New York: Dodd, Mead & Co.

—— (1970b) *Professional Dominance: The Social Structure of Medical Care*, New York: Atherton.

—— (1989) *Medical Work in America*, New Haven: Yale University Press.

Galbraith, J. K. (1956) *American Capitalism: The Concept of Countervailing Power*, Boston: Houghton Mifflin.

Glaser, W. (1993) 'The competition vogue and its outcomes', *Lancet* 27 March: 805–12.

Immergut, E. M. (1992) *Health Politics: Interests and Institutions in Western Europe*, New York: Cambridge University Press.

Jarausch, K. H. (1990) *The Unfree Professions*, New York: Oxford University Press.

Johnson, T. J. (1972) *Professions and Power*, London: Macmillan.

Jones, A. (ed.) (1991) *Professions and the State*, Philadelphia: Temple University Press.

Klein, R. (1990) 'The state and the profession: the politics of the double bed', *British Medical Journal* 3 October: 700–2.

Knox, R. (1993) *Germany's Health System: One Nation, United with Health Care for All*, New York: Faulkner & Gray.

Krause, E. A. (1988) 'Doctors, *partitocrazia*, and the Italian state', *Milbank Quarterly* 66 (Suppl. 2): 148–66.

Larkin, G. V. (1988) 'Medical dominance in Britain: image and historical reality', *The Milbank Quarterly* 66 (Suppl. 2): 117–32.

Larson, M. S. (1977) *The Rise of Professionalism: A Sociological Analysis*, Berkeley: University of California Press.

Leibfried, S. and Tennstedt, F. (1986) 'Social medicine vs professional dominance: the German experience', *American Journal of Public Health* 76: 78–83.

Light, D. W. (1979) 'Uncertainty and control in professional training', *Journal of Health and Social Behavior* 20: 310–22.

—— (1988) 'Turf battles and the theory of professional dominance', *Research in the Sociology of Health Care* 7: 203–25.

—— (1989) 'Social control and the American health care system', in H. E. Freeman and S. Levine (eds), *Handbook of Medical Sociology*, 4th edition, Englewood Cliffs, New Jersey: Prentice-Hall.

—— (1990) 'Bending the rules', *The Health Service Journal* 100: 1513–15.

—— (1991a) 'The restructuring of American health care', in T. J. Litman and S. Robins (eds), *Health Politics and Policy*, 2nd edition, New York: Wiley.

—— (1991b) 'Professionalism as a countervailing power', *Journal of Health Politics, Policy and Law* 16: 499–506.

—— (1991c) 'Effectiveness and efficiency under competition: the Cochrane test', *British Medical Journal* 16 November: 102–4.

—— (1993) 'Escaping the traps of postwar Western medicine', *European Journal of Public Health* 3: 223–31.

—— (1994) 'Comparative models of "health care" systems with application to Germany', in P. Conrad and R. Kern (eds), *The Sociology of Health and Illness*, 3rd edition, New York: St Martin's Press.

Light, D. W. and Levine, S. (1988) 'The changing character of the medical profession: a theoretical overview', *The Milbank Quarterly* 66 (Suppl. 2): 10–32.

Light, D. W., Liebfried, S. and Tennstedt, F. (1986) 'Social medicine vs professional dominance: the German experience', *American Journal of Public Health* 76(1): 78–83.

Light, D. W. and May, A. M. E. (eds) (1993) *Britain's Health System: From Welfare State to Managed Markets*, New York: Faulkner & Gray.

Light, D. W. and Schuller, A. S. (1986) *Political Values and Health Care: The German Experience*, Cambridge, Mass.: MIT Press.

Marmor, T. R. and Christianson, J. B. (1982) *Health Care Policy: A Political Economy Approach*, Beverly Hills: Sage.

Merton, R. K. and Barber, E. (1976) 'Sociological ambivalence', in R. K. Merton (ed.), *Sociological Ambivalence and Other Essays*, New York: Free Press.

Montesquieu, de S. C. L. (1748) *De l'Esprit des loix*, Geneva: Barillot & Sons.

Scott, W. R. (1993) 'The organization of medical care services: toward an integrated theoretical model', *Medical Care Review* 50: 271–304.

Starr, P. (1982) *The Social Transformation of American Medicine*, New York: Basic Books.

Steuart, J. (1767) *Inquiry into the Principles of Political Economy*, Vol. 1, London: Miller & Cadwell.

Stone, D. (1988) *Policy Paradox and Political Reason*, Boston: Scott, Foresman.

Waitzkin, H. (1983) *The Second Sickness: Contradictions of Capitalist Health Care*, New York: Free Press.

Walsh, D. C. (1987) *Corporate Physicians: Between Medicine and Management*, New Haven: Yale University Press.

Wilsford, D. (1991) *Doctors and the State: The Politics of Health Care in France and the United States*, Durham, NC: Duke University Press.

Part II

Health professions and the state in Britain

3 State control and the health professions in the United Kingdom
Historical perspectives

Gerry Larkin

Approaches to the analysis of professions in the general sociological literature and within medical sociology in the case of health professions share a linked limitation. In the former case there is a tendency in the broader academic discipline to consider professions, however in detail defined, as discretely bounded, successful occupations. This common assumption is then linked in the second case to a medico-centric bias, through an arguably understandable but disproportionate focus, in the United Kingdom at least, upon the medical profession. There are notable exceptions in the broader academic field to these initial remarks, evident for example most recently in the emphasis by Abbott (1988) upon the systematic interconnectedness of professions in their quest for jurisdictions of control. Within medical sociology, Stacey (1988) in particular locates her analysis of biomedicine firmly within the evolution of both the health-related and the broader social division of labour. However, despite these and other exceptions, our insights into the construction of expert labour have accumulated extensively through the study of 'end-process' occupational forms or outcomes. In particular, across the spectrum of health occupations an academic division of labour has also given separate and varied levels of attention to doctors, allied health professions and alternative practitioners rather than focused on the frameworks which inextricably link and shape their individual histories.

Whilst individual professions very often are held in view as end-states rather than in terms of the division of labour between them, some of the wider processes of attaining specific types of occupational power have none the less been cogently analysed. For example, the account by Johnson (1972) of oligarchic, collegiate and state-mediated stages of profession–client relationships emphasizes the variety of socio-historical contexts within which particular degrees of occupational power may develop or diminish. Freidson's approach, although less historically oriented than Johnson's, particularly links professional dominance in the medical sphere to control over the attendant division of labour (Freidson 1985). He does not, however, extensively comment on the conditions under which this kind of dominance is acquired rather than sustained. By contrast, Johnson (1982), through linking the emergence of the modern state and the transformation of collegiate-type professions, offers a way forward on this particular point. None the less, our understanding of these historical connections and their influence upon occupational formations is still at an early stage.

In general terms this chapter will argue that these and other analysts are correct in variously emphasizing the links between the context of occupational ascendancy and the character of professional power. In particular, however, the links between inter-occupational dominance and state formation need closer attention. These two dimensions, it will be argued, are constructed together, such that at least in the health field the professionalization of any one occupation must be viewed as part of a wider medico-bureaucratic shaping of the twentieth-century division of labour. This process is not a product of a predetermined state and medical profession, but rather is a dynamic alliance through which they have together established and renewed their earlier identities. The full ascendancy of medical professional power, beyond a collegiate or guild-based occupation in the marketplace, paradoxically has been an integral part of the transformation of the British state across the nineteenth and twentieth centuries. The broader case for reconsidering any assumption that professions and the state may be analysed separately is set out in chapter 1 by Terry Johnson.

Before turning to some historical detail to exemplify these points, some broad socio-historical differences should be noted between the United Kingdom and the United States, particularly given the shared character of their sociological literature. It has increasingly been recognized that the term 'profession', in its Anglo-American connotations, does not easily translate with the same meanings into other European languages and social contexts (Rueschmeyer 1983). In particular a principal expectation of separateness from the state has less validity in continental Europe where supervision by government is closer. Less recognized within a common language and academic literature is the relevance of some historical differences between Britain and America. These factors provided contrasting base-points for occupations which have attempted the transition to influence in their field in this century. For example, the nineteenth century American medical profession, after the deregulation period of Jacksonian democracy, consolidated its position in the marketplace against a less interventionist and stable central state authority. The westward expansion of the country, amongst other factors, created a distance between the central state and professional forms of organization, which should not be read into other contemporary contexts.

In the United Kingdom nineteenth-century government drew upon a longer centralized tradition of administration within which knowledge-based occupations were incorporated into the emergence of a modern bureaucracy. As the century developed, in medicine as with education and other areas, the state extended its mandate in partnership with a variety of managing groups and cadres. Thus the nineteenth-century proto-profession was transformed in this alliance from an interim collegiate mode of development to a new phase acting as an agent in the extension and reconstruction of the state itself. In this change of position its authority was not removed or reduced but rather redefined within the growing sphere of government. The collegiate mode, as identified by Johnson, involving control over clients within an expanding bourgeois class, as such secured no advance beyond that point as the forces and location of market expansion changed. As both bureaucratic and technological change intensified, occupational survival required a place within the expansion of state influence in health care.

THE MEDICO-BUREAUCRATIC COMPLEX

The transformation of the nineteenth-century profession and the extension of the state shelter are linked in the later conversion and reconstruction of the health care division of labour following earlier changes. The 1858 Medical Act, through statute placing the monitoring of educational and professional standards within the authority of a practitioner-dominated General Medical Council, may be seen to be a milestone in the confirmation of professional autonomy. However, the associated ending through this measure of the separate, albeit converging, castes of apothecary, surgeon and physician through the formation of a new occupational class, 'the registered medical practitioner', may be viewed otherwise. This new group and its members had a clarified identity as agents of the state in recording births, fitness, sickness and death. Unregistered practitioners could not certify statutory documents, could not receive fees for this work, and could not enter into the expanding public sector of medical care. The longer-term effects of state registration, converting *de jure* entitlements into a *de facto* monopoly of the bulk of practice, were of considerable significance (Waddington 1984). Statutory recognition for one type of practitioner hampered those without it, but this exclusive advantage only held any longer-term value through its broader conversion to a control of other occupations within the expanding state sector.

Through the nineteenth century most formal paid medical care had been delivered through solo practices. Hospital medicine in a modern form, with its attendant scale and structure of specialities, had yet to emerge, despite an accumulating range of insights which was to revolutionize medical practice. By the end of the nineteenth-century, however, a profession of practitioners mostly accustomed to individual patterns of working faced a number of challenges. Demand for medical care, partly in line with its enhanced effectiveness and growing safety, had increased. The state, prompted by ineffective *laissez-faire* policies, also had been drawn into the field of managing public health. A new organizational framework was required to deliver improved treatments in health care, beyond the few voluntary hospitals and the individualized medical market. A policy of expanding hospitals and clinics offered a way forward, but this development in turn required a complex labour force to sustain it. Neither the nineteenth-century profession nor the state at this point possessed a formula to manage the associated growing workforce. Rather, they shared a pre-existing relationship and a convergent interest in the ordering of the emerging division of labour.

This convergent project of control between profession and state over the enlarging arena of health work was linked to the subordination of newly emergent occupations, and the reinforced exclusion of others which had commenced in the nineteenth century. Subordination within the orthodox division of labour and the gradual convergence of medical and state power are discussed more extensively elsewhere (Larkin 1983). The first decades of the century saw the state regulation of midwives (1902), of nurses (1919), dentists (1921) and the containment of the professional aspirations of groups as diverse as physiotherapists and opticians. It is, however, perhaps the continuing exclusionary processes of non-recognized occupations up to the 1930s which more sharply point up the character of the joint medico-bureaucratic enterprise. State registration, however valuable, did not extend to the legal prohibition of health care offered by others. The medical profession thus remained dissatisfied with the common law rights of 'alternative' practitioners into the twentieth century, as evident in the *Report as to the Practice of Medicine and Surgery by Unqualified Persons in the United Kingdom* (HMSO 1910). The expansion of state services and the growing penalties of exclusion from them stimulated 'alternative' practitioners to join the new order, thereby challenging the link between the orthodox profession and state.

Medical professional opposition to the non-registered came to a strong point when influential doctors staffed the newly formed Ministry of Health after the First World War. The new Ministry was particularly dominated by its medical officers, who, as its official records indicate, were usually at one with their external professional colleagues on issues of occupational privilege. Medical herbalists, for example, with an ancient professional pedigree, were amongst the first to challenge the medical–Ministry alliance, to seek some benefit from inclusion in the new order. Their quest in reality was for a restoration of previously gained state favour, in that in the reign of Henry VIII their predecessors had secured advantages over the medical adversaries of their day. At that time the Company and Fellowship of Surgeons of London were held to have abused their powers granted under an Act of 1512, which gave physicians and surgeons practice rights within seven miles of the City of London, when 'examined, approved and admitted' by the Bishop of London. In parenthesis deprofessionalization or a reduction in occupational privileges is not new to the medical profession, as a correcting Act of 1542 indicates which redefined and reduced previous rights:

[Although] the most part of the persons of the said Craft of Surgeons have small cunning yet they will take great sums of money, and do little therefore, and by reason thereof they do often-times impair and hurt their patients, rather than do them good. In consideration whereof, and for the ease, comfort, succour, help, relief, and health of the King's poor subjects, inhabitants of this realm, now pained or diseased, or that hereafter shall be pained or diseased: Be it ordained, established, and enacted, by authority of this present Parliament, that at all time from henceforth it shall be lawful to every person being the King's subject, having knowledge and experience of the nature of herbs, roots, and waters, or of the operation of the same, by speculation or practise, within any part of the realm of England, or within any other the King's dominions, to practice, use, and minister in and to any outward sore, uncome wound, apostemations, outward swelling or disease, any herb or herbs, ointments, baths, pultess, and emplaisters, according to their cunning, experience, and knowledge in any of the diseases, sores and maladies beforesaid, and all other like to the same, or drinks for the stone, strangury, or agues, without suit, vexation, trouble, penalty, or loss of their goods; the foresaid statute in the foresaid third year of the King's most gracious reign, or any other act, ordinance, or statutes to the contrary heretofore made in anywise, notwithstanding.

(Public Record Office MH58: 106)

Following the Nurses' and Dentists' Acts of 1919 and 1921, in 1923 the Association of Medical Herbalists, perhaps naïvely, sought to restore and update these ancient prerogatives through Parliament. This attempt was dismissed by senior Ministry officials examining their draft bill as being 'most mischievous'. The bill proposed a Herbalists' Council to oversee their training and registration, with no provision, as in the case of the other Acts cited above, for oversight by representatives from the medical profession. Its intention, in Ministry perceptions if not reality, was to seek a share in 'all the rights of qualified medical practitioners', thus opening the way to their dispersal amongst other occupational claimants unwilling to accept a subordinate status. In particular herbalists wanted remuneration for treatment offered under the Insurance Acts, in other words to practise under the umbrella of state-sponsored provision. Their claims, and a further bill blocked in 1926, were rejected on the grounds that 'the state ought not to recognize any form of medical practice carried on by persons who have not received an adequate medical training'. The dispute continued through the 1920s until in 1932 the herbalists discovered that what they regarded as their correspondence with the Minister of Health in fact was being passed on to the General Medical Council to advise the Ministry of Health, and in turn released to journals of the pharmacy profession to stimulate its opposition in addition to that of the medical profession (Public Record Office MH58: 106).

This behaviour led to parliamentary questioning of the Minister, Sir Hilton Young, in 1932, regarding his department's impartiality in the regulation of health occupations. Although he was obliged somewhat lamely to respond that confidentiality had not been requested by herbalists in their dealings with the Ministry, in reality the General Medical Council was treated by its officials as another department of the state. In this period it was routinely involved in regulating groups outside its own immediate jurisdiction, under a fictional status as a source of extra-governmental advice (Larkin 1983). In reality its powers were considerably advanced beyond those of an advisory capacity, not least through its authority to remove from its register any doctor who worked with an unrecognized practitioner of any kind. Medical sensitivities to any kind of professional encroachment were still very considerable at the time, as the case of Herbert Barker, a successful lay practitioner, confirmed in 1932. Barker threw down a gauntlet to his critics, offering to demonstrate his skills in manipulation to leading medical specialists. Dr A. Cox, drawn into the controversy on behalf of the British Medical Association, argued in the correspondence columns of *The Times* (21 September 1932) that the fundamental issue was not Barker's competence. It was rather that recognizing it risked the whole structure of official training sustaining doctors, lawyers, veterinary surgeons, dentists and many others.

This hyperbole in argument, perhaps odd in its insecurity if the argument here of a mutual reinforcement of state and medical power is correct, was not unusual and indeed mild compared to that surrounding the osteopathic 'invasion' of the 1920s and 1930s. However, the medico-bureaucratic project principally depended upon relationships in one part of the state apparatus, which in broader terms should not be regarded as unitary or coordinated in operation. In particular the introduction of private members' bills in Parliament was an area of instability for the medical–Ministry alliance. As Sir George Newman, the Chief Medical Officer at the Ministry, wrote to Sir Donald Macalister, then president of the General Medical Council, of the first bill for state registration of osteopaths in 1931, there was 'no insuperable obstacle to the bill's ordinary progress through Parliament as an approved measure'. The latter's support was solicited to protect 'the integrity of medicine' against this eventuality. The finer details of osteopathy's challenge to the medical–Ministry alliance are discussed elsewhere (Larkin 1992), and only some principal features will be noted here. Unlike the case of herbalists and other alternative practitioners, osteopathy was an organized foreign import which had made some progress in securing recognition as a legitimate form of practice in the different conditions of the United States. Then, as perhaps today, although small in numbers, it was a relatively cohesive professional group in a world of medical sects. Its challenge, however, lay not so much in a different philosophy of healing, or concepts of pathology and treatment at variance with conventional medicine. It was rather that any recognition of these differences on a basis of professional equality threatened the integrity and cohesion of the medical profession–state relationship. Newman, like most of his professional colleagues, was opposed to any dilution of the privileges derived for the profession from the 1858 Act. This was presented or indeed seen not as self-interested behaviour, but as a joint venture in responsibly raising standards of provision for the public out of the harmful range of unauthorized practice.

Arrangements were made through government whips to block the bill, which surfaced again in the less easily managed House of Lords in 1934. Despite the vigorous opposition of the medical peers, or perhaps in part because of their arguments, the bill was referred to a select committee for further debate. Some peers were less concerned with Lord Moynihan's characterization of the bill, on behalf of his profession, as an 'endeavour to destroy the Hippocratic unity of medicine', and as only worthy of 'the derision of all competent and experienced minds', than the reported skills of osteopaths in treating hunting, polo and cricket injuries. In fact the medical–Ministry position was not based simply on excoriation, as briefing notes for the Minister of Health indicate in 1935. What would have been acceptable, these argued, was a position within which 'the registered medical practitioner . . . is fully responsible for diagnosis and treatment and the osteopath is a technician possessed of special manipulative skills whose responsibility is limited to carrying out manipulative work under the direction of his principal' (Public Record Office MH58: 107). Thus the fundamental issue was not therapeutic incompatibility, or scientifically informed as against fanciful practice, but authority and exclusivity as expressed through arguments cast in those terms. This was evident in Sir Henry Brackenbury's evidence to the ensuing Select Committee on behalf of the British Medical Association, which suggested that osteopathy had a considerable albeit limited usefulness, but only when subordinated to medical control. Sir Henry raised the further spectre of two separate classes of practitioner being present in every medical situation if the bill proceeded in its intended form. These arguments were reinforced by Sir Arthur Robinson, on behalf of the Ministry, who predicted a claim on the part of osteopaths to have the same position in the public services, such as the infectious disease service or the national insurance service, as the medical practitioner. In addition the Registrar-General pointed to a likely confusion of official medical certification processes, and eventually under the weight of this opposition the Committee reported adversely.

On a Ministry suggestion a voluntary rather than statutory register was established, but the longer-term consequence for alternative medicine was considerable. Most immediately the Ministry of Health refused any support for the British Osteopathic Association's appeal for establishing a hospital in London. The Chief Medical Officer advised the Minister against any assistance, lest 'sooner or later' on a new basis osteopaths would again press for state registration. They were excluded from the Emergency War Service, and favourably disposed doctors who valued their skills were encouraged instead to use physiotherapists who fully accepted or at least endured a subordinate status. However, the most lasting effect, indeed for all heterodox groups, was exclusion from the planning for and subsequent operation of the National Health Service. As a preface to this exclusion, the 1939 Cancer Act prohibited the non-registered from offering to treat cancers, whilst the 1941 Pharmacy and Medicines Act placed restrictions on practitioners other than doctors in treating a number of conditions, ranging from Bright's disease, cataracts and diabetes to epilepsy and tuberculosis. As Vaughan (1959) points out in his history of the British Medical Association, these measures represented an eventual success for the profession's decades-long campaign against quack practice and the commercial exploitation of bogus remedies.

For others, under the guise of public health precautions a dubious medical monopoly was being enforced with a growing intensity. In response in 1945 the first meeting of the British Health and Freedom Society was held. The Society claimed 11,000 members and a role as a united front for osteopaths, naturopaths, herbalists, anti-vaccinationists and others. Beveridge's plans were perceived as yet a further threat to their livelihoods, whence their claim that the compulsion on all citizens to contribute to the new national insurance scheme should be matched by state support for their choice of orthodox or unorthodox treatment.

As one complainant put it to Aneurin Bevan, the postwar socialist Minister of Health, even the doctors in the Labour Party are orthodox in their prejudices against other healing arts. Bevan's position, perhaps fortified by a need to avoid further provoking already inflamed opposition from some doctors to his plan to extend state provision, was the same as his predecessors. The 'floodgates' argument was produced, within which if any group other than doctors were to be recognized in the new National Health Service it would be impossible to know where to draw the line between herbalists, osteopaths, Christian Scientists and any other unorthodox forms of practice and, by implication, 'quackery' (Public Record Office MH77: 59).

CONCLUSION

Within the management of the division of labour, the above picture does not assume a complete and continuing harmony of viewpoint, but rather an important unity of project across several formative decades. It also does not assume an immutable relationship between both parties, but rather suggests that an understanding of the past terms of emergence of the medico-bureaucratic order may assist in appreciating its possibly transitory or evolving character. In many other respects through this period government policies and those of medical professional organizations have been at repeated variance. Many broader changes over recent decades both encompassing and within health care systems have had an effect on historical relationships. To touch on just a few, for example as Perkin (1989) argues, state professionals have been in retreat from the assault of market professionals seeking to capture the state apparatus for their particular ends. Linked fiscal crises of the state, emphases upon consumerism, more perhaps publicly jaundiced perceptions of experts or scientists, the 'return' of the market, albeit through state control as discussed in later chapters, may all be mentioned also. More directly in the health field, a widening appreciation of the limits to biomedicine, of the continuing recalcitrant character of chronic illnesses, and of enhanced expectations of the medical encounter may be of notable importance (Berliner 1984). Against the growth of such factors the past ascendancy of orthodox medicine may look less secure and extensive. Thus it can be asked whether the joint profession–state project has now run its course, or, as may be more likely, whether it is entering another and more pluralistic phase.

The 1980s and 1990s, after a period of earlier quiescence, have resembled the 1920s and 1930s, in an apparent resurfacing of debates concerning 'alternative' medicine. In the United States osteopathy, for example, may be in a process of partial incorporation into orthodox medicine (Baer 1981), whilst there are signs of fundamental realignments here in the United Kingdom. The King's Fund (1991) *Report of a Working Party on Osteopathy* pointed to significant changes in influential medical circles, certainly when measured against the Report on alternative medicine by the British Medical Association (1986). The former Report confidently asserted that both the public and the medical profession have over the years come to recognize osteopathic treatment as a valuable complement to conventional medicine. The British Medical Association was cited as now accepting that an organized, respectable and cohesive body of knowledge underlies osteopathic practice. The Report went on to make a case for state registration much as in the bitterly opposed bill of half a century previously, but this time against a claimed likely consensus between osteopaths, the main medical associations and the major political parties. On a closer reading, this indicated change of position, perhaps induced by a host of wider factors making orthodox medicine vulnerable, has limits.

The apparently path-breaking Report explicitly disavowed any support for osteopathic practice within the National Health Service. In other words the proposed regulation was of an occupation operating without restriction up to this point in the private commercial sector of health care, unlike orthodox medicine, which benefits from both public and private practice. It is of course possible that, following the ensuing state registration of osteopaths in 1993, any subsequent continuing exclusion from employment in state services will not be sustainable over time. However, if this change in access to state services occurs, it may not necessarily imply the end of the medico-bureaucratic order in one sense but rather its extension. The terms of state recognition have not challenged the organizing principles of the conventional medical division of labour but rather accepted their embrace. Osteopaths, as previously with dentists, nurses, midwives and the professions supplementary to medicine, have established a defined niche for themselves as specialist bio-mechanical manipulators. Previous claims to an equality of professional status and scope of practice to doctors have been abandoned in exchange for state registration.

In essence the medico-bureaucratic order, in this case as in others, can alter its scope, and in time is dynamic in both conserving and changing its position. Whilst earlier in this century the transformation of a nineteenth-century occupation and the extension of state sponsorship in health care merged in the control of the division of labour through exclusion and subordination, these circumstances to some degree have passed. The state no longer is limited to a choice of one managing agency as previously at the century's start, and within an established elaborate bureaucratized order medical monopolies in their various manifestations may be seen to be part of contemporary problems rather than vehicles for their resolution. In fact the medical–Ministry alliance has been displaced, with notable intensity of late, not so much by alternative medicine but by the new occupational class of manager, the custodians of cost control and performance measurement. Thus one state professional class, as the state further constructs itself, may be sharing influence with another, termed by Alford (1975) as corporate rationalizers, in a process as yet far from complete in outcome. This new type of alliance, emergent with state attempts to contain the cost of services, is based upon several internally competitive partners. At present, however, it is part of a growing pluralism in occupational control that is unclear in outcome, rather than any very radical redefining of the fundamental character of the medico-bureaucratic complex.

REFERENCES

Abbott, A. (1988) *The System of Professions: An Essay on the Division of Export Labor*, Chicago: University of Chicago Press.

Alford, R. (1975) *Health Care Politics*, Chicago: University of Chicago Press.

Baer, H. (1981) 'The organisational rejuvenation of osteopathy: a reflection of the decline of professional dominance in medicine', *Social Science and Medicine* 15A: 701–11.

Berliner, H. (1984) 'Scientific medicine since Flexner', in J. W. Salmon (ed.), *Alternative Medicines*, London: Tavistock.

British Medical Association (1986) *Report of the Board of Science and Education on Alternative Therapy*, London: BMA.

Freidson, E. (1985) 'The reorganisation of the medical profession', *Medical Care Review* 42(1): 11–35.

HMSO (1910) *Report as to the Practice of Medicine and Surgery by Unqualified Persons in the United Kingdom*, London: HMSO.

Johnson, T. J. (1972) *Professions and Power*, London: Macmillan

—— (1982) 'The state and the professions: peculiarities of the British', in A. Giddens and G. Mackenzie (eds), *Social Class and the Division of Labour: Essays in Honour of Ilya Neustadt*, Cambridge: Cambridge University Press.

King's Fund (1991) *Report of a Working Party on Osteopathy*, London: King's Fund Institute.

Larkin G. V. (1983) *Occupational Monopoly and Modern Medicine*, London: Tavistock.

—— (1988) 'Medical dominance in Britain: image and historical reality', *The Milbank Quarterly* 66 (Suppl. 2): 117–32.

—— (1992) 'Orthodox and osteopathic medicine in the inter-war years', in M. Saks (ed.), *Alternative Medicine in Britain*, Oxford: Clarendon Press.

Perkin, H. (1989) *The Rise of Professional Society*, London: Routledge.

Public Record Office *Ministry of Health Files* 58: 106, 107; 77: 59.

Rueschmeyer, D. (1983) 'Professional autonomy and the social control of expertise', in R. Dingwall and P. Lewis (eds), *The Sociology of the Professions*, London: Macmillan.

Stacey, M. (1988) *The Sociology of Health and Healing: A Textbook*, London: Unwin Hyman.

Vaughan, P. (1959) *Doctors' Commons*, London: Heinemann.

Waddington, I. (1984) *The Medical Profession in the Industrial Revolution*, Dublin: Gill & Macmillan.

4 Restructuring health and welfare professions in the United Kingdom

The impact of internal markets on the medical, nursing and social work professions

Andy Alaszewski

In the twentieth century a close alliance has developed between the state and the professional complex. The state has fostered the development of professionals, especially those involved in social welfare, and provided substantial funding for the activities of these professions. In exchange professionals have allocated state funding by identifying appropriate forms of client need and allocating resources to meet that need. The inexorable rise of state expenditure on welfare and the recessions of the 1980s have placed a strain on the relationship between the state and professionals. In the United Kingdom, the general election in 1979 resulted in the formation of a Conservative government heavily influenced by the rhetoric of the New Right and hostile to the public sector and public expenditure. The desire to reduce public expenditure has resulted in a substantial restructuring of the relationship between the state and professionals with the introduction of greater competition and the development of internal markets where full markets were not feasible. This chapter examines the ideological and practical background to this process and illustrates the developments by focusing on the changes in three professional groupings, the medical profession, nursing and social work.

PROFESSIONALS AND THE DEVELOPMENT OF STATE WELFARE

In the postwar period a political consensus developed about the role of the state in the relationship to the welfare of its citizens. In Britain the two major parties accepted that:

- certain citizens, for instance people who were either elderly, disabled or unemployed, could not compete in the market and therefore should receive state protection in the form of specific services and income support; and that
- certain services, such as health and education, could not be allocated justly and fairly by the market and therefore should be directly provided and allocated by the state.

The professions were central to this system of allocating resources. They played a key role in identifying those citizens who required services and in allocating the resources provided by the state. The welfare state was a 'professional state'.

Rhodes has described the postwar period as the 'era of the professional' (1987: 101).

This system of state funding allocated by professionals was seen as not only socially just but also economically efficient. Professionals had the confidence of citizens so were accepted as neutral agents for the just allocation of public resources and they had the technical expertise and specialists to allocate and utilize public resources efficiently. Talcott Parsons described the suitability of the professions for allocating resources in terms of their 'collectivity-orientation' and characterized it, in contrast with the self-interest of the businessman operating in the market, in the following way:

> the physician is a technically competent person whose competence and specific judgements and measures cannot be competently judged by the layman . . . it would be particularly difficult to implement the pattern of the business world (for the delivery of medical care), where each party to the situation is expected to be oriented to the rational pursuit of his own self-interests, and where there is an approach to the idea of 'caveat emptor'. In a broad sense it is surely clear that society would not tolerate the privileges which have been vested in the medical profession on such terms.
>
> (Parsons 1951: 463)

For this reason Parsons argued that medical care cannot be delivered within a market and that medical practitioners cannot behave as if they were in a market, for example by competing with each other.

> [The] collectivity-orientation of the physician is protected by a series of symbolically significant practices which serve to differentiate him sharply from the businessman. . . . The general picture is one of sharp segregation from the market and price practices of the business world, in ways which for the most part cut off the physician from many immediate opportunities which are treated as legitimately open to the businessman.
>
> (Parsons 1951: 464)

Parsons argued that the development of the professional complex had created a new form of social structure that was displacing political authoritarianism associated with the state and capitalistic exploitation associated with the market:

> It [the professional complex] has displaced the 'state', in the relatively modern sense of that term, and, more recently, the 'capitalistic' organisation of the economy. The massive emergence of the professional complex, not the special status of capitalistic or socialistic modes of organisation, is the crucial structural development in twentieth-century society.
>
> (Parsons 1966: 545)

THE CONSERVATIVES AND THE PROFESSIONALS

In the postwar period in Britain, many right-wing politicians, such as Winston

Churchill, were reluctant collectivists. They did not see any politically and intellectually viable alternative to the establishment of the welfare state. However, some right-wing academics such as Hayek and Friedman developed a theoretically grounded critique of the welfare state and outlined an alternative strategy. They challenged many of the basic assumptions of the welfare state. They argued that state protection of certain citizens made these citizens dependent on the state and destroyed their ability to care for themselves. Hayek warned of the dangers of collective political power:

> What is called economic power, while it can be an instrument of coercion, is in the hands of private individuals never exclusive or complete power, never power over the whole person. But centralised as an instrument of political power it creates a degree of dependence scarcely distinguishable from slavery.
>
> (1944: 43)

These critics argued that the removal of certain services from market provision created collective power. Individuals could only acquire services through state bureaucracies and became dependent on those bureaucracies and the professionals that staffed them. Professionals played a key role in creating and maintaining a dependency culture. Through their close relationship with the state, these professional created a monopoly in which they controlled not only the supply but also the demand for welfare services. Individuals could no longer plan and control important aspects of their lives because professionals had taken over the diagnosis of problems and the prescription of solutions. Individual wants were redefined by professionals as 'a need for a service' (Culyer 1976: 14; Illich 1976).

The solution advocated by these critics involved returning control and responsibility to individuals through the re-establishment of a market in professional services. Lees described the advantages of the market for allocating health care in the following way:

- 'The market is generally superior to the ballot box as a means of registering consumer preferences.'
- 'Medical care is a personal consumption good, not markedly different from the generality of goods bought by consumers.'
- 'Therefore, if the aim is to maximize consumer satisfaction, medical care should be supplied through the market' (1964: 14).

These right-wing critics remained relatively marginal and peripheral to the main debates about the development of the welfare state and the role of professionals until the 1970s. During that decade the relationship between professionals and the state came under stress. Economic fluctuations placed considerable stress on public finance. The state found it increasingly difficult to control overall welfare expenditure, especially as professionals took successful actions to raise their own incomes. At the same time the freedom of professionals to allocate state funds with minimal accountability appeared to create problems of both efficiency and social justice. Professionals were inefficient as they allocated resources to modes of service delivery that were of high cost and apparently less effective than cheaper alternatives. In the health service the problems related to the continued expansion of hospital-based high-technology medicine associated with the neglect of more cost-effective aspects of medicine, for example general practice and preventative medicine, and that of less glamorous client groups and services often referred to as Cinderella services, for instance services for older and for handicapped people. In social services the problems related to the continued expansion of residential accommodation, particularly for elderly people. The social justice issue related to the continued persistence of geographic and social inequalities, especially of resource inputs.

The various stresses in the 1970s were associated with the development of the concept of ungovernability, that is, that government in social democratic societies was uncontrollably increasing in size and scope so that it was no longer possible to exert complete administrative control and in particular to coordinate the activities of different parts of the government machine. These parts operated autonomously and often in conflict with each other. This feeling of ungovernability was associated with the large-scale restructuring of the machinery of government that took place in the United Kingdom in the mid-1970s. In the 1960s the Labour government had initiated a series of reviews of different parts of the government machine, including central government, local government and the National Health Service. These reviews led to a series of restructuring in the 1970s that created large administrative units and agencies in central and local government. These welfare agencies were designed to facilitate the introduction of corporate managerial processes and to draw professionals into the process of management and resource allocation. These new agencies had been conceived in the 1960s when the accepted view was that there would be a continued expansion of the resources allocated to welfare. However, they became operational in the 1970s during a period of fiscal crisis; indeed they contributed to the crisis by adding to the rapid expansion of public service costs.

In 1979, the Conservative Party led by Margaret Thatcher was elected to government in a time of crisis, following a period of industrial action in the public sector referred to as the 'winter of discontent'. The Conservative Party was committed to addressing the crisis of government by 'rolling back the frontiers of the state'. It intended to reduce the size and scope of government by exposing as many areas of life as possible to the rigours of market forces. Nigel Lawson, one of Thatcher's close associates, described the changes in the following way:

> The rehabilitation of market forces in the early 1980s was seen at first as an aberration from the postwar consensus, and one that was likely to be short-lived. But I have no doubt that, as a longer-term perspective develops, history will judge that intervention and planning were the aberration, and that the market economy is the normal healthy way of life.

> (quoted in Riddell 1989: 208)

Initially the main focus of attack was the public sector itself and in particular public expenditure not the professions *per se*. The new administration tempered ideology with pragmatism (see Flynn 1989; Hudson 1989). The principles of the New Right were first applied to organizations and agencies that did not enjoy public support or were weak. For example, the powers and rights of trade unions and local authorities were restricted through a series of laws. Similarly within agencies such as local government and the National Health Service, certain groups, mainly manual workers, were exposed to the rigours of market forces through the process of competitive tendering. Established professional groups such as doctors were protected from the rigours of the market. In the health service a division was made between support services (and staff), that is, manual workers, which were exposed to market forces, and clinical services (and staff), that is professional workers, which were not. Some 'weaker' professional groups were more closely involved in this first phase, for example opticians were rapidly exposed to the full rigour of market forces (Higgins 1988), and the government engaged in a long-drawn-out battle with school teachers over pay and the control of the school curriculum.

It was only in the Conservative government's third term of office that the political agenda shifted from the control of public expenditure to the specific process of allocation and financial control and the key role played by professional groups in it. This role has now moved to the top of the political agenda. The government has sought to change it, and has attempted to alter its own relationship with these established professional groups in a number of ways, namely through:

• the establishment or improvement of market mechanisms and the increase of financial control;
• the reduction in restrictive practices to 'create a level playing field';
• increases in the power and status of consumers, especially by increasing the flow of information to potential consumers;
• inspection of the quality of services.

The precise form in which these established professions are being exposed to market forces has depended on their existing relationship to the market. Although there is an extremely limited market in medical services and the majority of medical services are funded and provided by the state through the National Health Service, the medical profession has maintained a semi-autonomous position as seller of services to the National Health Service. This ambiguous position is now being exploited with moves towards a state-funded or 'internal market' in health care. Social work is most closely tied to the state provision of services. There is virtually no private market in social work services and almost all social workers are fully integrated into the state provision of welfare either in local authority social services departments or in probation services. Only the voluntary sector remains autonomous, but even this is heavily reliant on the state for funding. The changes associated with the development of child care and community care will have a major impact on the nature of social work practice and it is possible to identify mechanisms for introducing market forces into social services.

THE MEDICAL PROFESSION

In the twentieth century, the medical profession in the United Kingdom has developed a partnership with the state to provide comprehensive health care, free at the point of delivery. This relationship has developed slowly, even hesitantly, and the medical profession has often tried to resist closer relations (see Honigsbaum 1979 and Macdonald 1988). The profession has been divided into three main sections that have enjoyed different status and autonomy and have developed relationships with the state in different ways. Public health doctors developed in the nineteenth century as close agents of the state in the implementation of public health measures and in the development of public health services especially within the framework of local government. The formation of the National Health Service in 1948 eroded the power and status of public health doctors and the reorganization of the National Health Service in 1974 destroyed their local authority power base and left them searching for a role. General practitioners accepted state funding through the insurance system introduced before the First World War and were incorporated in a semi-detached manner into the National Health Service in 1948. Hospital consultants, especially in the voluntary hospitals, guarded their autonomy jealously and only accepted incorporation into the National Health Service in 1948 on favourable terms.

The incorporation of different parts of the profession into the National Health Service has been a compromise in which the medical profession is seen as enjoying many of the benefits of a close relationship with the state, for example, guaranteed high incomes and access to facilities, with few of the disadvantages. In the case of general practitioners this can be seen in their peculiar employment status. In some respects, general practitioners are like small businessmen who contract to sell medical services to the state, that is, they maintain a high level of autonomy, but they also share some of the benefits of employee status, such as guaranteed state-funded pensions (see Maynard 1989). The medical profession utilized resources provided by the state but did not accept any accountability for the use of these resources. For example, Stacey argued that by 'Insisting on [the] principle of clinical autonomy in 1974, the [medical] profession avoided the managerial control which was imposed upon all other health care professionals in the NHS' (1989: 13). Clinical autonomy can be defined as the freedom to define the needs of patients and to use National Health Service resources to meet these needs.

Market mechanisms and financial control

The New Right has been hostile to the political and economic privileges of the medical profession and has tended to view the National Health Service as 'a monopoly or a monolith which impedes innovation' (Bosanquet 1983: 150). However, there are serious problems in replacing the National Health Service with a free market in health care. Not only does the National Health Service enjoy considerable public support but it is also a means of achieving government objectives, such as cost control and equity of resource allocation. The solution to this problem has been to move to 'internal markets' in health care. Bevan defines internal markets in the following way:

> [The] the government would distribute resources financed by taxation to agencies responsible for providing health care to defined populations by capitation [as now]; the difference from current arrangements is that these agencies would seek to maximise benefits from health services for their defined populations from their allocation by buying services from suppliers who would compete on quality and price.
>
> (1989: 53)

In 1987, after a particularly bruising debate with the Opposition over the funding of the National Health Service during which she had to sacrifice John Moore, her Secretary of State for Social Services, the Prime Minister, Mrs Thatcher, decided to chair a comprehensive review of the funding of the National Health Service. The results of this review were published as a Government White Paper on the National Health Service, *Working for Patients* (Department of Health 1989d), and subsequently implemented as the National Health Service and Community Care Act (1990).

This Act created the framework for an internal market in health care. In this market there is a clear division between purchasers, who will receive state funding, and producers, who will contract to sell their services to the 'purchasers'. Patients are not defined as 'purchasers' – although citizens who are over 60 who will receive a subsidy (tax-relief) if they contract to buy services from the private sector (Department of Health 1989d: para. 9.9). General practitioners can apply to be fundholders, that is, to act as 'surrogate' consumers by claiming a budget for services and using this budget to 'purchase' hospital services for their patients. Initially the main 'purchasers' will be District Health Authorities, who will be responsible for purchasing hospital and community services for all the residents of their district. They will eventually receive a weighted capitation budget based largely on the population profile of their district (Department of Health 1989d: paras 4.8 and 4.11) and will prepare a purchasing plan to obtain the service which their Director of Public Health has defined as necessary in his or her evaluation of the health needs of the district's population. The development of contracting alters the rationing process in the National Health Service. Prior to contracting, all services which doctors believed could meet medical needs were funded. In the contracting services only those services are provided for which there is an explicit contract.

The reduction of restrictive practices

The government proposes that 'fundholding' general practitioners and purchasing authorities will be able to purchase services from a range of competing producers. Thus a District Health Authority will be able to purchase services from hospitals it continues to manage directly, from hospitals directly managed by other District Health Authorities, from private hospitals and from hospital trusts. The hospital trust represent a major innovation. The government is blurring the divide between private and public provision by allowing a hospital or equivalent unit to achieve self-governing status (see Department of Health 1989d and the National Health Service and Community Care Act 1990: chapter 3, paras 5–11). The new National Health Service trusts in some respects represent a return to pre-National Health Service voluntary hospitals. The National Health Service trusts will own their own hospitals, employ their own staff and compete in the market for patients.

The government is creating the framework for an internal market in health care, in which there will be a free flow of patients and funding to reward quality and value for money and a 'level playing field' between different providers. The basis of this market will be contracts. Details of the contracting process are quite complex and have been the subject of a special working paper (Department of Health 1989a). The relationship between purchasers and providers of services will be structured through contracts or management budgets. The management budget will be 'structured as contracts but will be enforced through the normal management process' (Department of Health 1989a: para. 2.1). The relationship between 'purchasers' and 'providers' will be based on an agreement between the two parties which will specify the nature of the service and type of payment but can take different forms according to different circumstances.

Consumers and information

At the same time as the government is increasing pressure from above through restructuring funding arrangements, it is also exerting increased pressure on the medical profession from below by enhancing the power of patients. The government is doing this by clearly specifying the rights of patients through *The Patient's Charter* and by enhancing the flow of information so that patients can exert pressure on their medical practitioners.

The Patient's Charter is the National Health Service's version of the *Citizen's Charter* and is the first comprehensive statement of patients' rights and the standard of service which professionals are expected to provide. Several of the ten specified rights have direct implications for medical professionals. For example, the Charter specifies that the rights of individual users are as follows:

- 'to be given a clear explanation of any treatment proposed, including any risks and any alternatives, before you decide whether you will agree to treatment';
- 'to have access to your health records, and to know that those working for the NHS are under a legal duty to keep their contents confidential' (Department of Health 1991b: 9).

Similarly some of the National Charter Standards will also influence practice. For example:

- Waiting time in outpatients clinics. 'The Charter Standard is that you will be given a specific appointment time and be seen within thirty minutes of that time.'
- Cancellation of operations. 'The Charter Standard is that your operation should not be cancelled on the day you are due to arrive in hospital' (Department of Health 1991b: 14).

As part of the process of increased accountability, medical practitioners will have to provide more information about their activities and these will be subject to greater scrutiny. Information is the basis of the market. For example, if general practitioners are to act as 'surrogate' consumers and act on behalf of their patients, then it is essential that 'patients must be able to exercise a real choice between GPs' (Department of Health 1989d: para. 7.4). To exercise this choice patients need information about the services of different general practices and need to be able to use this information by easily changing their general practitioner. Although many general practitioners accept that it is 'good medical practice . . . to provide patients with a booklet describing basic information about a practice' (Thompson 1989: 65), there has been resistance within the profession to advertising and to the free movement of patients between practices. As Titmuss (1958) pointed out, the free movement of patients between practices was restricted by a reluctant Ministry of Health in 1950 to satisfy general practitioners who claimed that some patients made excessive changes of doctor. The government 'believes that the advertising of services offered by practices should be the norm' (Department of Health 1989d: para. 7.5) and has persuaded the General Medical Council to relax its restrictions so that information can be provided in public information centres such as libraries (though not in the press). The government has also removed most of the administrative impediments that prevented patients moving easily from one practice to another.

Quality

The concern with improving and using information can also be seen in the move towards medical audit. One of the dangers of a market system in which services are specified in terms of quantity is that producers may reduce quality. The medical profession has been aware of wide and unacceptable variations in the standards and quality of practice and has set up its own peer review mechanisms (see Royal College of General Practitioners 1985). The government proposes to build on the various peer review mechanisms by developing a comprehensive system of medical audit and linking it into the management and contract processes of the National Health Service. Thus each health agency will have to establish an audit advisory committee or group and all consultants and general practitioners will be required by their new job descriptions or conditions of service to participate in the auditing process. The information will then be used in a variety of ways; for example, it can be used as part of the contracting process (Department of Health 1989b).

Impact on medicine

The proposals for the health service involve not only the creation of an internal market in health but also a major change in the relationship between the state and the medical profession. The medical profession has established a position of almost unique privilege. It has had access to major state resources without experiencing the pressure to account for the use of these resources. The New Right endorses the current government proposals as a pragmatic move to reduce state control and planning, to increase consumer choice and introduce the discipline of the market. For example, Marsland, writing in *The Salisbury Review*, describes the government proposals in the following way: 'One might imagine, to judge from the self-righteous hysteria provoked in the health establishment by the Government's modest and cautious proposals, that the NHS was beyond improvement. . . . It is a health consumer's charter' (1989: 8–9).

The changes are likely to have a differential impact on different sections of the medical profession. Public health doctors have a clear role and status in the new system as providers of information and guardians of quality. There is a great opportunity for general practitioners to enhance their control. If they become budget-holders, they will control the process of resource allocation in the National Health Service. If they do not, then the power will shift to managers in the purchasing authorities and 'it will be the responsibility of the GP to ensure that the patient's referral is covered, or can be covered by an appropriate contract or non-contractually' (Department of Health 1989a: para. 3.1).

Hospital specialists are potentially squeezed the most. If they remain in directly managed units, then:

> Ministers therefore consider it essential that District Managers should have a clear understanding of the work which is being undertaken by consultants and would be in a position to make changes following discussions with them. In other words, there is a need for an improved process of accountability. . . . The Government does intend that [consultant's contracts] . . . should be managed locally.
>
> (Department of Health 1989c: paras 2.1–2.2)

If they opt out, then they will depend on the patients and contracts which they can attract from purchasers.

The proposals will mean that the medical profession maintains access to increasing amounts of public resources but it will have to compete and/or account for them. The profession's money, power and prestige are being challenged (Hafferty 1988) and it appears relatively powerless to stop the changes.

NURSING

Within the National Health Service, doctors form the élite decision-making group. They have been at the centre of the reform debate. Although nurses form the single largest group of National Health Service employees, that is, 405,280

Whole Time Equivalents or 50.9 per cent of the total workforce (Department of Health 1991a: C16), they have been far more peripheral to the debate about change. Indeed in the key White Paper, *Working for Patients* (Department of Health 1989d), nurses are conspicuous by their absence. However, as the Audit Commission (1991: 2) point out, 'Nursing is too important a component of patient care and of hospital budgets to be left to develop in isolation', and nursing is also undergoing radical restructuring.

Market mechanisms and financial control

Although the medical profession remains the major allocator of resources within the National Health Service, increasing emphasis is being given to nurses as financial controllers. This can be most clearly seen in the shift from ward sisters to ward managers with an increasing emphasis on the financial and managerial role of senior ward nurses.

Traditionally power and status in nursing was concentrated within the hierarchy of nurse managers. Successive reforms in the 1980s have resulted in a considerable reduction of the size, power and control of the nursing hierarchy (Harrison 1988: 146–9) and a shift of responsibility to ward level. In the new National Health Service trusts, nursing budgets are being delegated to ward level. Ward managers are given budgets which indicate the amount of money being allocated to the ward for nursing staff and associated expenditure and the expenditure of the ward under these budgets' heads. The ward manager is expected to control some items such as payment for additional staff and is given some freedom about the particular skill mix and therefore expenditure patterns on his or her ward. Ward managers do not have the same power and authority to challenge nursing budgets as senior nurse managers. Thus the shift of responsibility to ward managers is being accompanied by an increase in control by general managers over nursing budgets.

Reduction of restrictive practices

In nursing terms this means a fundamental change in the organization and management of nursing work with an extended role for clinical nurses and a shift from functional to primary nursing.

Traditionally nurses operated very much as assistants to doctors; doctors diagnosed and prescribed and nurses carried out these prescriptions. There is an increasing emphasis on a distinctive nurse role that is complementary to but independent from the doctor's role, that is, a unique nursing process in which nurses identify and treat the individual needs of each patient. This process is concerned with the physical and mental well-being of the patient and his or her ability to perform the activities of everyday living (see Beardshaw and Robinson 1990).

In the nursing process the role of the nurse is to assess the patient on admission, plan the patient's everyday care, monitor the patient's progress and prepare for his or her discharge. This care planning is complementary to and supports the doctor's main activity of diagnosing and prescribing treatment for the patient's underlying medical condition. Each patient has a nursing care plan that forms the basis of that patient's care from admission to discharge.

The development of a clear role and technology for nursing reduces restrictive practices so nurses can take on some of the activities of doctors and pass more routine and menial tasks to support workers. One of the few references to nursing in *Working for Patients* is made in this context:

> There have been many developments in recent years in the better use of nursing staff, but the Government believes that there is still scope for more progress at local level. . . . As part of this initiative, local managers, in consultation with their professional colleagues, will be expected to re-examine all areas of work to identify the most cost-effective use of professional skills. This may involve a reappraisal of traditional patterns and practices. Examples include the extended role of nurses to cover specific duties normally undertaken by junior doctors in areas of high technology care and casualty departments; the use of clerical rather than nursing staff in receptionist work.
>
> (Department of Health 1989d: para. 2.13)

Consumers and information

The Patient's Charter (Department of Health 1991b) specifies that each patient has the right to have a named nurse. The concept of a named nurse has major implications both for accountability and for the organization of nursing. Patients admitted to hospital in the United Kingdom come under the medical care of a named medical specialist or consultant. The development of a named nurse makes it clear that the consultant is only responsible for the medical care of the patient; the named nurse is responsible for the separate and distinctive area of nursing care, for keeping patients and their relatives informed and for the standard of care.

This personal responsibility has organizational implications. Traditionally work on wards was task-oriented, that is, there was a routine of nursing tasks such as waking and washing the patients and these tasks were shared between all the nurses on each shift. These tasks were allocated by the senior nurse at the start of each shift. The introduction of the named nurse undermines the task-allocation of nursing duties and reinforces the development of patient-centred care which is called either team or primary nursing (Black 1992). Each of two or three named nurses on a ward is responsible for planning and delivering the care for her or his patients.

Quality of services

Nursing has taken on increasing responsibility for the quality of services. There have been two parallel developments, accountability and standards. The professional validating body, the United Kingdom Central Council for Nursing,

Midwifery and Health Visiting, has issued guidelines which make it clear that all qualified nurses are responsible for the quality of services received by patients. The United Kingdom Central Council has issued a code of conduct to all qualified nurses which specifies that all qualified nurses:

shall act, at all times, in such a manner as to

- safeguard and promote the interests of individual patients and clients;
- serve the interests of society;
- justify public trust and confidence; and
- uphold and enhance the good standing and reputation of the profession.

(1992: 2)

These underlying aims are given substance by sixteen standards that specify the ways in which nurses are expected to discharge their professional duties. Most of the standards relate to the ways in which nurses should discharge their responsibilities to patients. For example, to maintain professional standards nurses must 'recognise and respect the uniqueness and dignity of each patient and client, and respond to their need for care, irrespective of their ethnic origin, religious beliefs, personal attributes, the nature of their health problems or any other factor' (United Kingdom Central Council 1992: 3).

The United Kingdom Central Council code of practice provides a clear statement of public expectations of the ways in which nurses will discharge their professional responsibilities and defines the ways in which each nurse is accountable for her or his actions. This personal responsibility is linked to the development of quality assurance procedures and the development of clear and explicit standards.

The role of nurses, especially ward managers, in setting and maintaining standards is a major theme in the review by the Audit Commission (1991) of ward nursing. The Commission's report argues that quality can be assessed using a number of measures including 'patient perceptions, easily quantifiable indicators . . . and assessment of the ways nursing care is delivered and the ward environment' (1991: para. 15). The Commission's report gives ward nurses the lead role in identifying and improving quality but *subject* to the overall control of managers:

Much of the detailed work on improving quality should be led by ward nurses themselves using quality *assurance* structures and procedures. . . . But periodic quality *assessment* is also necessary if managers are to fulfil their duty of ensuring that basic standards of nursing care are not neglected. It helps mangers to identify underlying reasons common to a number of wards, some of which may be outside the power of individual wards to correct.

(1991: para. 16)

Impact on nursing

Although nursing has traditionally enjoyed a relatively high social status in the United Kingdom, this status has been mainly associated with senior members of the profession, such as senior hospital or health authority nurse managers. Front-line workers have enjoyed relatively little autonomy, being subject to close control by either their own senior managers or by medical staff. Nurses have been accountable for the care they provide, but in a task-allocation system tasks were divided and shared between groups of nurses, so accountability was often diffused amongst this group.

The current changes offer a great opportunity to front-line nurses. They are having to accept increased personal accountability for their actions, but in exchange they are receiving increased autonomy. The nursing process offers them a clear and distinctive technology for assessing needs and planning and delivering patients' nursing needs that can enhance the autonomy and independence of patients and speed their recovery and discharge from hospital.

SOCIAL WORK

In many respects the changes to social work are both the greatest and the most surprising. When the Conservative Party was elected to government in 1979, it was extremely hostile to social work. Many in the Party saw social work as a bastion of both municipal socialism and the dependency culture. The Secretary of State for Social Services imposed a 10 per cent cut on the budget of social services departments and initiated a review of the role of social workers (Barclay 1982). As the Conservative Party enters its fourth term of office the situation has changed completely: a former social worker, Virginia Bottomley, has been appointed as Secretary of State for Health, resources are to be shifted from the social security budget to the social services and there are major new roles for social workers.

In social work there is no overall review equivalent to the National Health Service review but there have been specific reviews of community care and children's services that taken together add up to the most fundamental change in social services organization and social work practice since the 1940s.

The most radical change is also the most difficult to document. It is in many ways implicit. The major review of social services in the 1960s, the Seebohm Report (1968), envisaged a generic social work profession providing a range of services to a diversity of clients. The current proposals involve an implicit restriction – the main clients of social services will be the vulnerable and dependent who need special protection, in particular children who are at risk, people with learning difficulties, physical disabilities and mental illness and certain groups of elderly people. This restriction can be seen in the Community Care White Paper in which government states that two of the key components of community care are:

- 'services that intervene no more than is necessary to foster independence'; and
- 'services that concentrate on those with the greatest need'

(Department of Health and Department of
Social Security 1989: para. 1.10)

Similarly the 1989 Children Act also limits the intervention of social services to specific identifiable areas:

> The welfare of the children is primarily the parents' responsibility and the state should help parents discharge their parental responsibilities when necessary, but otherwise not intervene. Equally, in the public domain, the state should only intervene in cases where the children are 'in need'. The definition of 'in need' is open to quite broad interpretation but it is nevertheless intended to limit the remit of state intervention in family life.
>
> (Family and Child Care Law Training Group 1989: 9)

Market mechanisms and financial control

In some ways the 1989 Children Act and the community care proposals build upon and reinforce different traditions within social services and social work. The Children Act is based on the professional child care tradition and places emphasis on the social workers' role in protecting children, acting as advocates and participating in legal proceedings. The community care proposals are more related to the traditions of the old welfare departments, with an emphasis on the social workers' role in allocating limited resources and administering services. This is also reflected in the different genesis of the two sets of proposals. The Children Act originated in continuing concern about the development of children's services within local authority social services departments, particularly the apparently never-ending procession of child abuse inquiries. The community care proposals originate with concerns about the growth of social security funding of private sector residential accommodation and a search for methods of capping this demand-led expansion.

However, there are important underlying similarities in the proposals for child care and community care and parallels with the development of the National Health Service. It is argued by the government that the two are inextricably linked:

> The two programmes are consistent and complementary and, taken together, set a fresh agenda and new challenges for social services authorities for the next decade. There is no intention of creating a division between child care and community care services; the full range of social service authority functions should continue to form a coherent whole.
>
> (Department of Health and Department of Social Security 1989: para. 1.3)

It is possible to see some social workers developing a 'surrogate' consumer role as purchasers of services on behalf of their clients. This can be seen in the 'care management' role. In the community care proposals: 'the Government sees considerable merit in nominating a "care manager" to take responsibility for ensuring that individuals' needs are regularly reviewed, resources are managed effectively and that each service user has a single point of contact' (Department of Health and Department of Social Security 1989: para. 3.3.2). The government clearly sees the Kent Scheme (Challis and Davies 1986) as a model and envisages care managers should manage and deploy resources on behalf of their clients in a devolved budgetary system (Department of Health and Department of Social Security 1989: para. 3.3.5.)

In the Children Act the new care procedures effectively create a care management role. Under the new Act there is 'one route into care, whichever court hears the case' (Family and Child Care Law Training Group 1989: 23), and a care order places upon the local authority 'parental' responsibility for ensuring a child is adequately cared for and protected. The local authority can discharge its responsibility in a variety of ways and therefore can choose the most appropriate care package. Effectively field social workers will become care managers developing individually tailored packages of services to promote the care of children and prevent the breakdown of family relations.

The reduction of restrictive practices

The second parallel with the health service review is the definition of a distinctive group of workers as service providers who will be expected to compete with providers from other agencies and from the independent sector. Within the community care proposals there is an explicit commitment to a flourishing independent sector. Although the government has decided not to extend 'compulsory competitive tendering to social care services' (Department of Health and Department of Social Security 1989: para. 3.4.7) it clearly expects local authorities to make maximum use of the independent sector (para. 1.2) and expects local authorities to 'make greater use of service specifications, agency agreements and contracts' (para. 3.4.7) not only for residential services but also for domiciliary, day and respite care (para. 3.4.4). The government expects local authorities to promote a mixed economy of social care by:

- 'determining clear specifications of service requirements, and arrangements for tenders and contracts';
- 'taking steps to stimulate the setting up of "not for profit" agencies';
- 'identifying areas of their own work which are sufficiently self-contained to be suitable for "floating off" as self-managing units';
- 'stimulating the development of new voluntary sector activity'

(para. 3.4.6).

In the Children Act there is also an emphasis on the development of a mixed economy with local authorities using and cooperating with a range of services. For example, the Children Act places a duty on local authorities to 'facilitate the provision by others (including in particular voluntary organizations) of services which the authorities have power to provide' (Children Act 1989: 17(5)(a)). These services include day care, accommodation, advice and assistance.

Consumers and information

The ability of clients such as children and frail elderly people to identify and express their interest is often limited. Therefore the case managers take on the role of advocate and their assessments are part of the crucial process of identifying clients' real needs (see Barker *et al.* 1989: 1504). The Children Act places a specific duty on local authorities to undertake proper assessment and to act as advocates for children in need. The London Training Group emphasizes the general importance of assessment and its specific importance in relationship to child protection: 'The duty [in the Act] to identify children in need will require assessments, according to agreed criteria within local authorities such assessments should form the basis for service provision' (Family and Child Care Law Training Group 1989: 20).

In the community care White Paper there is also a concern with assessment but the emphasis is more on the efficient allocation of resources than on client advocacy.

> The aim of assessment should be to arrive at a decision on whether services should be provided and in what form. . . . The new assessment arrangements will involve significant changes in the way professional workers are expected to operate.
>
> (Department of Health and Department of Social
> Security 1989: paras 3.2.12 and 3.2.13)

As in the health service reforms, there is a strong emphasis on the improved availability and use of information. This can be seen in the emphasis on assessment and the strengthening of inspection powers. In the health service reforms, information is seen as a resource which will enable patients to make informed choices about issues such as the selection of general practitioners. In the social services reforms, choice and individual preferences are also stressed. For example, in the Children Act a court is required 'to have particular regard to the ascertainable wishes and feelings of the child concerned' (Children Act 1989: 1(3)(a)). Similarly there is a shift in attitude to parents, emphasizing their rights to information and their rights of appeal and complaint.

Quality

The other aspect of collection and use of information is the all-pervading concern with quality. In the Children Act the government acknowledges the current limitations of inspection and monitoring and proposes not only to modernize and rationalize the law on standards of private care (Department of Health and Social Security 1987: Foreword), but also to apply the same processes to services currently administered by local authorities.

Although the government is not establishing a separate ministry nor an independent inspectorate of residential care, it proposes that all forms of residential care will be under the scrutiny of independent inspection units. These will be 'expected to apply the same quality assurance criteria to all homes' (Department of Health and Department of Social Security 1989: para. 5.19) and should include inspectors recruited from outside social services departments (para. 5.20). On a national level there will be increased monitoring of local authorities to ensure the policy is developed in line with national policies with an enhanced role for the Social Services Inspectorate (para. 5.25).

Impact on social work

The changes amount to a radical restructuring of social work. The proposal will mean that additional resources will flow into social services departments and that social workers will have a clearly defined role in allocating them. Care managers will have increased flexibility to manage packages of resources but they will have to account for their use of these resources. In theory they will be advocates for clients and therefore accountable to them, but in practice as gatekeepers they will experience increasing accountability to management. Social work will be explicitly split between service purchasers (care managers) and service providers (residential and day-care workers). A division has always existed between field-workers who formed the trained élite and residential and day-care workers who formed the untrained bulk of service providers. The proposals will formalize this division and place the effective power in the hands of the care managers and their equivalents.

CONCLUSION

Current changes in the United Kingdom mark an important development in the relationship between a variety of welfare professionals and the state. These changes are neither simple nor straightforward. They do not represent a simple increase of state power over professional groups with a movement towards a status as state bureaucrats. Indeed in both the National Health Service and social services the moves towards incorporating the professionals in the bureaucratic hierarchy have been reversed. The rhetoric is not that of the state bureaucracy but that of the private sector and business. Yet at the same time the state has sought to increase its control over the total level of resources and the ways in which they are allocated. Market mechanisms are utilized but both professional groupings and individual professionals are left with choice on how they fit into the market.

The medical profession has attempted to retain some of the benefits of a market position but has sought to protect itself from the competitive aspects of the market. The current reforms of the health field offer medical professionals a clear choice. They can either become 'players' in an internal market or they can accept 'managerial protection' at the cost of some autonomy.

Within nursing a major shift in power is taking place. The power, status and roles of ward nurses is being enhanced, especially with the development of the new technology of nursing and of the ward manager role. Ward nurses are being given a lead role in financial control, enhancing consumer rights and promoting quality. The dependence of ward nurses on senior nurse mangers and doctors is being eroded but is being replaced with increased control and scrutiny by general managers.

The social work profession has traditionally been part of the administration and provision of welfare. In some respects social workers are facing similar pressure. They are being 'offered' professional status if they are willing to participate in and even operate a market system. If social workers do not accept the responsibilities of managing resources, then other groups will take on this role.

REFERENCES

Audit Commission (1991) *The Virtue of Patients: Making the Best Use of Ward Nursing Resources*, London: HMSO.
Barclay, P. (1982) *Social Workers: Their Tasks and Roles*, London: Bedford Square Press.
Barker, L., Peck, E. and Smith, H. (1989) 'Safeguarding service users', *The Health Service Journal* 7 December: 1502–4.
Beardshaw, V. and Robinson, R. (1990) *New for Old? Prospects for Nursing in the 1990s*, London: King's Fund Institute.
Bevan, G. (1989) 'Reforming UK health care: internal markets or emergent planning?', *Fiscal Studies* 10: 53–71.
Black, F. (1992) *Primary Nursing: An Introductory Guide*, London: King's Fund Institute.
Bosanquet, N. (1983) *After the New Right*, London: Heinemann.
Challis, D. and Davies, B. (1986) *Case Management in Community Care*, Aldershot: Gower.
Culyer, A. J. (1976) *Need and the National Health Service*, Oxford: Martin Robertson.
Department of Health (1989a) *Funding and Contracts for Hospital Services, NHS Review*, Working Paper 2, London: HMSO.
—— (1989b) *Medical Audit, NHS Review*, Working Paper 6, London: HMSO.
—— (1989c) *NHS Consultants: Appointments, Contracts and Distinction Awards, NHS Review*, Working Paper 7, London: HMSO.
—— (1989d) *Working for Patients*, London: HMSO.
—— (1991a) *NHS Workforce in England*, London: HMSO.
—— (1991b) *The Patient's Charter*, London: HMSO.
Department of Health and Social Security (1987) *The Law on Child Care and Family Services*, London: HMSO.
—— (1989) *Caring for People*, London: HMSO.
Family and Child Care Law Training Group (1989) *Training Together: A Training and Curriculum Model for the Children Act 1989*, London: Family and Child Care Law Training Group, London Boroughs' Training Committee and London Boroughs' Children's Regional Planning Committee.
Flynn, N. (1989) 'The "New Right" and social policy', *Policy and Politics* 17: 97–109.
Hafferty, F. W. (1988) 'Theories at the crossroads: a discussion of evolving views on medicine as a profession', *The Milbank Quarterly* 66 (Suppl. 2): 202–25.
Harrison, S. (1988) 'The workforce and the new managerialism', in R. Maxwell (ed.), *Reshaping the National Health Service*, Hermitage, Berks: Policy Journals.
Hayek, F. (1944) *The Road to Serfdom*, London: Routledge.
Higgins, J. (1988) *The Business of Medicine*, London: Macmillan.
Honigsbaum, F. (1979) *The Division in British Medicine: A History of the Separation of General Practice from Hospital Care, 1911–1968*, London: Kogan Page.
Hudson, B. (1989) 'Impact of the New Right', *The Health Service Journal* 14/28 December: 1546–7.
Illich, I. (1976) *Limits to Medicine: Medical Nemesis: The Expropriation of Health*, Harmondsworth: Penguin.
Lees, D. S. (1964) 'Health through choice', in Institute of Economic Affairs (ed.),

Monopoly or Choice in Health Services? Contrasting Approaches to Principles and Practice in Britain and America, Institute of Economic Affairs, Occasional Paper No. 3.

Macdonald, K.M. (1988) *Professions and the State*, Occasional Papers in Sociology and Social Policy No. 16, Department of Sociology, University of Surrey, Guildford.

Marsland, D. (1989) 'An appreciation of the NHS review', *The Salisbury Review* 8: 8–10.

Maynard A. (1989) 'From an ivory tower', *The Health Service Journal* 12 October: 1252.

Parsons, T. (1951) *The Social System*, London: Routledge & Kegan Paul.

—— (1966) 'Professions', in D. L. Sills (ed.), *International Encyclopedia of the Social Sciences*, Vol. 12, New York: Macmillan & the Free Press.

Rhodes, R. A. W. (1987) 'Mrs Thatcher and local government: intentions and achievements', in L. Robins (ed.), *Political Institutions in Britain: Development and Change*, London: Longman.

Riddell, P. (1989) *The Thatcher Decade*, Oxford: Blackwell.

Royal College of General Practitioners (1985) *Quality in General Practice*, Policy Statement 2, London: Royal College of General Practitioners.

Seebohm Report (1968) *Report of the Committee on Local Authority and Allied Personal Social Services*, London: HMSO.

Stacey, M. (1989) 'The General Medical Council and professional accountability', *Public Policy and Administration* 4: 12–27.

Thompson, M. K. (1989) 'Hypothesis: old people would benefit from a patient-held standardized primary heath care record', *Age and Ageing* 18: 64–6.

Titmuss, R. M. (1958) *Essays on The Welfare State*, London: Allen & Unwin.

United Kingdom Central Council (1992) *Code of Professional Conduct*, 3rd edition, London: UKCC.

5 Shifting spheres of opportunity

The professional powers of general practitioners within the British National Health Service

Judith Allsop

This chapter examines the key health policy changes in the 1980s in the British National Health Service. The aim is to assess the impact on the professional powers of an important sub-group, general practitioners. Although the medical profession is often treated as homogeneous, the circumstances in which different groups of doctors practise affects the degree of autonomy they exercise and the extent to which they dominate in various spheres and relationships. The chapter examines the work-world of general practitioners and how the changing practices of government have brought shifts in the general practitioner's relationships with the state, professional colleagues and patients. It is argued that the professional autonomy of the general practitioner has been enhanced by the introduction of market forces and general practitioners have gained in relation to their hospital colleagues. The state has gained political advantage by focusing on divisions of interest within the profession.

The chapter first outlines the theoretical stance taken in relation to the analysis of professional power. It looks briefly at the state/professional relationship in general and then at the specifics of general practice within the National Health Service. The health service reforms of the 1980s and early 1990s are described and their impact on general practitioners considered.

ANALYSES OF PROFESSIONAL POWER

Writers on the professions have engaged in a debate about the relative decline or maintenance of professional dominance. Those who take a broadly Marxist perspective have suggested professional decline under pressure from capitalism. It is argued that doctors have become 'proletarianized': their work routinized and their decision-making controlled by corporations and state regulation (McKinlay and Arches 1985; McKinlay and Stoeckle 1988; Haug 1988).

Others, such as Freidson (1985), Larkin (1988), Elston (1991) and Moran and Wood (1993), have argued the case for continuing medical dominance. Elston (1991) gives a clear account of aspects of medical dominance. She separates social and cultural authority from professional autonomy. Social authority is defined as medicine's commands over the actions of others in the division of labour, and cultural authority as the prevalence of medical definitions of reality in judgements involving health and illness. Professional autonomy, on the other hand, is the term used to refer to the legitimated control which the occupation exercises over its organization and terms of work. Elston concludes that while there have been challenges in the 1980s, nevertheless, social and cultural authority and professional autonomy remain strong.

Moran and Wood in a comparative study of Germany, Britain and the United States, argue: 'everywhere doctors are under pressure, but everywhere they have power' (1993: 136). The pressures derive from the concerns of government in capitalist societies. Governments are concerned to cut health service expenditures, to curtail the demand for services and obtain value for money. Also, there are pressures which derive from the increasing size of the arenas in which doctors work or are employed. This tends to increase the management function. However, Moran and Wood argue that doctors' power remains in the system of state-licensed self-regulation; in governments' inability to control entry to the profession; and the pay of doctors and the control over clinical work. Due to the monopoly over medical knowledge and the ability to give an authoritative interpretation of the individual case, doctors continue to dominate essential areas and decisions.

Political analysts of British medicine, perhaps because the National Health Service is more centralized and bureaucratically controlled, have focused on arenas of relative professional and state dominance. They have drawn attention to the countervailing powers of government and the profession in the policy process and their dependence on each other. In this chapter, the particular case of general practitioners and the National Health Service reforms will be examined. While acknowledging that the state and the profession have particular spheres of concern and relative autonomy, I shall argue that recent policy shifts which aim to promote primary care and introduce market forces have freed general practitioners from some constraints, although they have imposed others. There have been clear shifts in the practices of government. The institutions which define spheres of relative autonomy remain largely untouched but the introduction of the rules of the market game have brought changes in behaviour and gains to those in a position to exploit them.

GENERAL PRACTITIONERS AND THE NATIONAL HEALTH SERVICE

It has already been pointed out that the British system of health care is highly centralized. Government controls the size of the National Health Service budget which provides most health care. The cost of health care in Britain is relatively low and some contributing factors are the low physician/patient ratio and the emphasis on providing services at primary care level through the general practitioner (OECD 1992). General practitioners and their ancillary staff both treat patients and act as gatekeepers to specialist hospital and community care. Almost half of the doctors working in the National Health Service are general practitioners, and there are almost twice as many general practitioners as doctors at consultant grade in the hospital service (NAHAT 1993). In 1992, the share of the National Health Service devoted to the family practitioner services was about 24 per cent, of which expenditure on family doctors was 34 per cent and the drugs they prescribe 36 per cent. In recent years, expenditure on these aspects of the service has been growing, although there have been a number of measures to control prescribing (Taylor 1991; Audit Commission 1993).

General practitioners are also a key professional group in the functioning of the modern welfare state. Their role goes beyond dealing with the sick and acting as gatekeeper to more expensive hospital care, to include the certification of unfitness for work and the assessement of disability benefit. They can also influence access to other benefits such as housing. The vast majority of the population, 98 per cent, are registered with a National Health Service general practitioner and on average people visit their general practitioner about four times a year (General Household Survey 1993).

In common with the medical profession as a whole, general practitioners have benefited from the social and cultural authority accorded to medical work and from the institutions which limit competition and provide self-regulation. The state has regulated pay through a national negotiating machinery. This aimed to provide the general practitioner with a target income agreed between the state and the profession. The state has also controlled strictly the distribution of general practitioners throughout the country in the interests of equity. However, within these parameters general practitioners have considerable autonomy in how, and with whom, they work. They were, and are, a powerful structured interest group well represented at national level through the British Medical Association with an effective network of local committees. These can bring matters of local concern quickly on to the national agenda. General practitioners have considerable job security. Until 1990, when it was set at 70, there was no statutory retirement age.

In many ways, general practitioners had made a favourable bargain with the state. Up until the mid-1980s, there was virtually no knowledge about, or scrutiny of, the day-to-day work of general practitioners apart from some monitoring of prescribing from peers or others. The type of practice, who was employed, the decisions made about treatment and care, were matters for individual decision and judgement and general practitioners did not have to consider the financial consequences of their clinical decisions to refer. Indeed, their most crucial role was as gatekeeper to the hospital. In Britain, the only other access to the specialist is through an Accident and Emergency department.

Although there were local-level organizations, the Family Practitioner Committees, from 1990, called Family Health Service Authorities, which managed the contracts of general practitioners, these exercised little influence, let alone control (Allsop and May 1986). The small scale of general practitioner practice, its diversity and the nature of medical work made this intrinsically difficult. In sum, general practitioners had considerable professional autonomy in day-to-day work, although they had a relatively low status as compared to the hospital doctor and were less integrated into a network of professional associations. Moreover, general practitioners' patients have been slow to exercise a 'voice' in relation to the service received and the lack of information has made 'exit' from one practice to another difficult. In effect, general practitioners have acted as small monopolistic suppliers of primary care as they have determined what was available and dominated the division of labour in the practice.

GENERAL PRACTICE AND HEALTH POLICY IN THE 1980s

The new liberalism

In 1980s Britain under Conservative governments, the ideology of neo-liberalism placed an emphasis on freeing the market to more competitive forces in both the private and public sectors. Within government, the aim was to privatize areas of the public sector; subject those which remained to internal competition; and draw on private sector management techniques to 'unbundle' larger organizations. Responsibility for meeting specified goals and managing within budgets was devolved downwards. Aspects of general strategy, regulation and monitoring remained at the centre. As Gamble (1988) suggests, Thatcherism as a political ideology aimed to achieve the twin goals of increasing competition and state regulation simultaneously. The policy was outlined in a 1988 Cabinet Office paper, *The Next Steps* (Efficiency Unit 1988).

Gordon comments on the way in which this process changes behaviour at the level of the individual:

> [The] liberal idea of government consists – over and above the economic market in commodities and services, whose existence forms the classical attribution of an autonomous rationality to the processes of civil society – in the form of something like a second order of governmental goods and services. It becomes the ambition of neo-liberalism to implicate the individual citizen, as player and partner, into this market game.
>
> (1991: 36)

It is argued here that general practitioners and their patients have been drawn into the market. This has been, first, through the policy shift towards primary and preventive care; second, through new forms of control associated with the internal market; and, third, through policies to make the consumer more active.

The shift towards primary care

From the mid-1980s onwards, primary care, and particularly general practice, moved up the government's policy agenda. This was motivated by cost considerations and the need to respond to the changing pattern of disease. There had been a drift towards more costly hospital medicine. It was believed that many procedures could be provided more cheaply and effectively from general practice. This was particularly so because the ageing population had brought more conditions where care and self-medication were more appropriate than hospital treatment. It was also argued that some serious illnesses could be prevented from developing by early intervention and health education. An example of the thinking of policy-makers was the report of the National Audit Office (1989), which recognized the very high rates of heart disease and some of the cancers in Britain compared to other European countries and the high cost of treatment to the economy. An earlier White Paper, *Promoting Better Health* (Department of Health 1987), had already outlined a role for general practice. Additional resources were to be available to encourage general practitioners to employ practice staff to carry out more health surveillance. In 1992, *The Health of the Nation* (Department of Health 1992a) laid out a national strategy for England with targets for the improvement of health status.

One of the stumbling blocks to changing primary care was the general practitioner's contract of employment which had been drawn up in the 1960s. In 1990, despite opposition from the general practitioners' negotiating body, a new contract (Department of Health 1989a) was introduced. It contained new requirements and controls which increased the powers of the authorities responsible for family practitioners, now renamed Family Health Service Authorities. General practitioners were now required to carry out activities to screen their practice populations for illness as well as treating it.

The most important aspects of the new contract were the requirements:

- to provide more data on practice activity for the Family Health Service Authorities and to produce annual reports;
- to prescribe within indicative prescribing budgets;
- to offer an annual home visit to patients over 75 and assess their needs;
- to offer a health check for new patients;
- to meet targets for vaccination, immunization and cervical cytology;
- to follow locally determined protocols if providing child health surveillance.

The Family Health Service Authorities had increased responsibility for monitoring activity, assessing whether targets had been met to qualify for additional payments and for allocating funds differentially to practices for staff, premises and computers. Family Health Service Authorities were also to appoint independent professional advisers to assist in monitoring practices and to encourage medical audit. In sum, surveillance of general practitioners' activity was increased and they were required to provide more services. The method of payment was changed to introduce financial incentives to carry out more medical work within the practice, such as minor surgery.

The 1990 NHS reforms

Working for Patients (Department of Health 1989b), the Prime Minister's review of the National Health Service, laid down a blueprint for introducing internal competition into the National Health Service. It was later enacted through the 1990 National Health Service and Community Care Act. Some measures had already been introduced to increase competition and 'fair trading' generally

(Miller 1992). For example, in 1988, the Monopolies and Mergers Commission recommended a liberalization of the rules over advertising. The General Medical Council, the profession's regulatory body, agreed to the production of practice leaflets and practices were asked to provide these for their patients. General practitioners could also provide information about their approach to medical practice to the public and the media.

The main consequence of the reforms is that a distinction is now made between those who purchase health services for their populations – the District Health Authorities, and those who provide services, the hospital and community trusts and the remaining minority of directly managed units. The District Health Authorities receive budgets based on population and other social variables. Contracts are placed with service providers who compete on the basis of price and quality.

General practitioners could influence the types of contracts by working with District Health Authorities to draw up the specifications or they could become general practitioner fundholders and place contracts for a limited range of services themselves. By 1991, general practitioners in practices with populations over 9,000 could opt to become fundholders to purchase certain hospital services such as elective referrals to hospitals, outpatient visits and diagnostic services. There was an additional allowance for prescribing, management and computing costs. From 1993, additional funds were made available to purchase community care services. The funding made available to general practitioner fundholders was deducted from the District Health Authorities budget at regional level.

There are clearly incentives for general practitioners to become fundholders in terms of autonomy as well as financially. Savings can be used to extend and improve practices and the patients of fundholding practices may receive favourable treatment as the provider is seeking income. Fundholders are proxy buyers on behalf of their practice and continue to hold a strong bargaining position on behalf of their patients (Hughes 1993). General practitioners who are not fundholders can also be involved in the purchasing process by expressing their views to purchasers through the Family Health Service Authorities or District Health Authorities, but the influence is less direct as it does not involve monetary transactions. Some general practitioners have developed alliances with other practices to increase their influence in the contracting process. So despite the loss of influence at Family Health Service Authority level as the number of doctors was reduced from eight to one, general practitioners have gained in other respects.

Activating the consumer

The third aspect of the health service reforms designed to produce a quasi-market has been through activating the consumer. Practices are expected to produce practice leaflets while Family Health Service Authorities are encouraged to find out what people want through surveys and consultation with local groups. The Citizen's Charter Initiative has led to the production of a variety of charters for public services. These include *The Patient's Charter* (Department of Health

1991), which outlined rights and standards of service and a charter specific to primary care (Department of Health 1992b). The charters stress the importance of providing information for people, setting performance standards, having a complaints procedure if things go wrong and a means of redress.

The changes proposed in the new contract and *Working for Patients* (Department of Health 1989b) were not initially welcomed by general practitioners. In 1989, there was bitter opposition in well-publicized media campaigns (Butler 1992). Day and Klein (1991) have argued this was in part due to the way in which the usual channels for negotiation between the profession and the state were by-passed. Changes were imposed through the parliamentary process in a manner reminiscent of the 1946 National Health Service Act.

However, by 1991, the overt opposition to government reforms had subsided and, despite the advice of their leaders in the British Medical Association, many general practitioners showed themselves eager to apply for fundholding status. By 1992, about 14 per cent of the population (285 practices) was covered by fundholding practices. By 1993, this had risen to 25 per cent (Audit Commission 1993). Among other general practitioners, many saw the financial advantages of the new contract and the greater flexibility and additional resources available through funding from the Family Health Service Authorities.

THE EFFECT OF THE REFORMS ON GENERAL PRACTITIONERS' OPPORTUNITIES AND PROFESSIONAL POWERS

In some respects, the National Health Service reforms have brought a clear increase in the control over, and the surveillance of, the work of general practitioners by the state. Additional data are required by the Family Health Service Authorities on aspects of patient activity. Annual reports must be produced and additional funds can be made contingent on providing business plans and improving practice management. The Family Health Service Authorities' potential for control, and that of other central bodies, has been aided by the availability of information technology. Computerized financial and patient activity systems enable the Family Health Service Authorities to chart the progress of practices. However, comparative information can also help general practitioners manage their practice. Information technology is itself a neutral tool. Currently, evidence suggests that Family Health Service Authorities have not yet developed a sufficiently clear view of their role to influence medical work. They lack the managerial capacity to control what goes on in the large number of small practices (Audit Commission 1993).

Increasingly, general practitioners themselves have invested in computers and many have used the technology to manage and develop work in their practices. In 1987, 10 per cent of practices had computers. By 1991, this had risen to over 60 per cent and is predicted to rise to 85 per cent by 1995. Not surprisingly, a higher proportion of the larger practices are computerized (Audit Commission 1993).

A further recommendation of *Working for Patients* was the appointment of professional advisers to give clinical advice as Family Health Service Authorities themselves lacked the expertise to assess standards of medical work. The recent Audit Commission report (1993) indicates that professional advisers have been used sparingly as they are expensive to employ. Those who have been appointed have tended to concentrate on advice on prescribing rather than aspects of diagnosis and treatment.

While the effect of new controls has been limited, the scale of practices in terms of staff employed has increased. For example, the numbers of practice nurses alone doubled between 1988 and 1990. Many more tasks are now undertaken by other health workers under supervision from the doctor. There is also evidence that more activity previously carried out in the hospital, such as out-patient clinics and minor surgery, is shifting to general practice (Boyle and Smaje 1992).

The scope of general practitioners' preventive work has also increased. There is evidence that government targets for screening have been met (Audit Commission 1993) and also that preventive work generates additional demand. For example, one study of annual health checks for elderly people found that 43 per cent had some form of unmet need (Brown *et al.* 1992). The consequence of this is an extension of the general practitioners' and other health workers' cultural authority over the well population. The purpose of screening is to detect those at risk of more serious illness so that they can be counselled about life-styles. As Armstrong (1983) argues in the *Political Anatomy of the Body*, population medicine is an extension of the clinical gaze into those who are well and therefore an extension of state control. Patient compliance is ensured through claims for the advantages of early detection. Doctor compliance is ensured by financial incentives. The efficacy of some screening is questioned by doctors themselves (Allsop 1990; Hann 1993).

In terms of their relationships with hospital doctors and their patients, general practitioner fundholders have clearly gained in both autonomy and influence. The study by Glennerster *et al.* (1992) of a sample of practices found a variety of innovations with doctors taking the initiative to develop their practice and to get a better service for their patients. Moreover, many general practitioners have made considerable savings in the first year of fundholding which could be ploughed back into their practices (Audit Commission 1993). General practitioner fundholders have been able to gain priority treatment for their patients as they bring additional income to trusts. The increase in fundholding is itself an indication of its popularity (Bain 1993).

While many general practitioners have proved to be adept at using the opportunities the market provides, others have lagged behind. For example, in 1991, a study of 2,000 practices found that 60 per cent did not prepare business plans; 20 per cent did not employ practice managers; and 64 per cent did not prepare budgets. Not even all general practitioner fundholders had a business plan (Quinn 1991). Leese and Bosanquet (1989) found an increasing bifurcation between the larger, well-managed practice often in a better-off area and the small practice in poor premises with a population ranked high on indicators of social deprivation. Market forces with easier movement of better informed patients are likely to exacerbate these trends.

For patients, the introduction of the market has brought greater inequalities as they remain relatively dependent on what their practice has to offer. The general practitioner continues to control medical knowledge and act as a gatekeeper. Patients are not often in a position to judge whether advice or treatment is appropriate. They usually assume competence. However, there are some signs that people who use the health service are becoming more active. For example, complaints about health care continue to rise. Moreover, current proposals to introduce practice-based complaints systems will increase general practitioner control over the complaint process (British Medical Association 1993).

Governments continue to apply pressure to open up the practices of medicine, and professional institutions themselves are becoming more visible, even if the pace is slow (Stacey 1992). The internal market itself is bringing a managerial focus on, and more knowledge about, the details of service delivery; what constitutes good practice and what services costs. So far, general practice has been relatively immune from the scrutiny being applied to hospital and community services. This may be due to general practitioners' position as potential purchasers as well as providers. It also reflects the nature of their work and their autonomy to practise.

CONCLUSION

This chapter began by examining the issue of professional dominance. It assessed the effect of changes in the practice of government on the position of the general practitioner in the wake of the health service reforms. I have argued that the reforms have provided opportunities for the general practitioner in a number of spheres – in relation to the scope of work; access to resources to improve services; the span of control over others; and in general practitioners' bargaining position with service providers. So far, because of the intrinsic difficulties of reviewing day-to-day practice and the weakness of Family Health Service Authorities, general practitioners have remained relatively immune from scrutiny, although their activity is more closely monitored. Ironically, the overall effect of introducing market forces into the National Health Service has been to allow the central state to step back. The 'invisible hand' of the market determines the behaviour of individuals in the health arena and the visibility of government's crucial role in funding is reduced.

REFERENCES

Allsop, J. (1990) *Changing Primary Care: The Role of Facilitators*, London: King's Fund Institute.
Allsop, J. and May, A. (1986) *The Emperor's New Clothes: Family Practitioner Committees in the 1980s*, London: King's Fund Institute.
Armstrong, D. (1983) *The Political Anatomy of the Body: Medical Knowledge in Britain in the Twentieth Century*, Cambridge: Cambridge University Press.
Audit Commission (1993) *Practices Make Perfect: The Role of the Family Health Services Authority*, Local Government Report No. 10, London: HMSO.

Bain, J. (1993) 'Budget holding: here to stay?', *British Medical Journal* 306: 1186–8.

Boyle, S. and Smaje, C. (1992) 'Minor surgery in general practice: the effect of the 1990 GP contract', in A. Harrison (ed.), *Health Care UK 1991*, London: King's Fund Institute.

British Medical Association (1993) *Evidence to the Wilson Committee NHS Complaints Review*, London: BMA.

Brown, K., Williams, E. and Groom, L. (1992) 'Health checks of patients 75 years and over in Nottinghamshire after the new GP contract', *British Medical Journal* 305: 619–21.

Butler,J. (1992) *Patient's Policies and Politics: Before and After Working for Patients*, Buckingham: Open University Press.

Day, P. and Klein, R. (1991) 'Political theory and policy practice: the case of general practice 1911–1991'. Paper given at the Conference of the Political Science Association, University of Lancaster, 15–17 April.

Department of Health (1987) *Promoting Better Health*, London: HMSO.

—— (1989a) *General Practice in the NHS: A 1990 Contract*, London: HMSO.

—— (1989b) *Working for Patients*, London: HMSO.

—— (1991) *The Patient's Charter*, London: HMSO.

—— (1992a) *The Health of the Nation*, London: HMSO.

—— (1992b) *The Patient's Charter and Primary Health Care*, EL (92)88.

Efficiency Unit (1988) *Improving the Management of Government: The Next Steps*, London: HMSO.

Elston, M. (1991) 'The politics of professional power: medicine in a changing health service', in J. Gabe, M. Calnan and M. Bury (eds), *The Sociology of the Health Service*, London: Routledge.

Freidson, E. (1985) 'The reorganisation of the medical profession', *Medical Care* 42(1): 11–33.

Gamble, A. (1988) *The Free Economy and the Strong State*, Basingstoke: Macmillan.

Glennester, H., Matsaganis, M. and Owens, P. (1992) *A Foothold for Fund Raising*, London: King's Fund Institute.

Gordon, C. (1991) 'Government rationality: an introduction', in G. Burchell, C. Gordon and P. Miller (eds), *The Foucault Effect: Studies in Governmentality*, London: Harvester Wheatsheaf.

Hann, A. (1993) 'The decision to screen', in M. Mills (ed.), *Prevention, Health and British Politics*, Aldershot: Avebury.

Haug, M. (1988) 'A re-examination of the hypothesis of physician deprofessionalisation', *The Milbank Quarterly* 66 (Suppl. 2): 48–56.

Hughes, D. (1993) 'Letting the market work?', in R. Page and J. Baldock (eds), *Social Policy Review* 5: 104–24.

Larkin, G. V. (1988) 'Medical dominance in Britain: image and historical reality', *The Milbank Quarterly* 66 (Suppl. 2): 117–32.

Leese, B. and Bosanquet, N. (1989) 'High and low incomes in general practice', *British Medical Journal* 298: 932–4.

McKinlay, J. B. and Arches, J. (1985) 'Towards the proletarianization of physicians', *International Journal of Health Services* 15(2): 161–95.

McKinlay, J. B. and Stoeckle, J.D. (1988) 'Corporatization and the social transformation of doctoring', *International Journal of Health Services* 18(2): 191–205.

Miller, F. (1992) 'Health policy, competition and professional behaviour', in A. Harrison (ed.), *Health Care UK 1991*, London: King's Fund Institute.

Moran, M. and Wood, B. (1993) *States, Regulation and the Medical Profession*, Buckingham: Open University Press.

NAHAT (1993) *NHS Handbook*, 8th edition, Tunbridge Wells: JMH Publishing.

National Audit Office (1989) *NHS Coronary Health*, London: HMSO.

OECD (1992) *The Reform of Health Care: A Comparative Analysis of Seven OECD Countries*, Paris: OECD.

Quinn, G. (1991) *The Management of General Practice*, Cranfield: Stoy Hayward Consulting and Cranfield School of Management.

Stacey, M. (1992) *Regulating British Medicine: The General Medical Council*, Chichester: John Wiley.

Taylor, D. (1991) *Developing Primary Care: Opportunities for the 1990s*, London: King's Fund Institute.

6 Doctors, peer review and quality assurance

Mike Dent

This chapter is concerned with the issues of medical audit and clinical budgeting within the hospital sector of the United Kingdom National Health Service and the implications this may have for the medical autonomy of hospital doctors. In the United Kingdom, the medical profession, at least until recently, has been able to counter any threats to its professional autonomy. Yet, with the current moves away from a welfare state model of health care and towards a more market-driven one, it may be that the profession will now be finally incorporated into the service class in an organic role as opposed to the traditional one they have tended to play previously (Abercrombie and Urry 1983: 147).[1] If this is so, then the situation will be unique in Europe in adapting, as it does, the United States system characterized by Freddi (1989: 13) as 'market efficiency coupled with liberty' as opposed to the 'solidarity coupled with equality' systems characteristic of Europe generally.

The central argument in this chapter will be that the state and the medical profession within Western capitalist societies are in a mutually ambivalent relationship. The institutional power and status enjoyed by doctors is largely the consequence of the commitment of governments to the provision of allopathic health care for the general population. At the same time, no government is able to ensure the provision of such services without the cooperation of the medical profession. Doctors, individually and collectively, predominantly control the system of medical education and training and the quality of medical care as well as the diagnosis of disease and the treatment of patients. No government in the West has found a way of usurping these responsibilities, although various attempts have been made to modify the ground-rules in order to control the cost of public sector health care.

This chapter is divided into four parts: first, an analysis of the organization of the medical profession; second, an account of changes in the hospital sector within the United Kingdom and an assessment of the influence of the American health maintenance organizational model; third, a discussion of medical audit, its introduction into the United Kingdom and the role it has played in inhibiting the development of clinical budgeting; fourth, a discussion of the role of the 'internal market' in transforming the debates and negotiations on medical audit within the United Kingdom. This is followed by the conclusions.

THE MEDICAL PROFESSION AND PROFESSIONAL AUTONOMY

It is in the public sector environment that we find the professions have developed a particularly distinct role. Without the market to dictate priorities directly it has been the professions, to a greater or lesser degree, which have been responsible for defining them. To some extent, this relationship between state and profession would appear to parallel that of responsible autonomy. Friedman (1977), in his modification of labour process theory, argues that one could usefully distinguish between two contrasting management strategies of managerial control. The first, direct control, corresponds with the notion of Braverman (1974), of managerial control typified by Taylorism and the assumption that management dictates, or attempts to dictate, all aspects of the work process. This is not the case with hospital doctors. The second strategy is termed by Friedman as responsible autonomy. As he says, this 'type of strategy attempts to harness the adaptability of labour power by giving workers leeway and encouraging them to adapt to changing situations in a manner beneficial to the firm' (1977: 78). This model is derived from the Tavistock Institute's socio-technical systems approach to job design (1977: 100–1). In the words of Friedman: 'To do this top managers give workers status, authority and responsibility ... [They] try to win their loyalty, and co-opt their organisations to the firm's ideal (... the competitive struggle) ideologically' (1977: 78). On the face of it, there are a number of parallels between responsible autonomy and professional autonomy – not least because the occupational groups thus organized are differentiated from other groups within the work organization on the basis of the central role they have within the division of labour. There is, nevertheless, a crucial difference between the two types of autonomies. In the case of the former the autonomy is the outcome of management strategies within a context of prevailing labour market conditions and worker resistance (Friedman, 1977). Whereas, by contrast, professional autonomy is the outcome of the strategies of organized occupational/professional groups that historically precedes the rise of monopoly capital (Johnson, 1972: 52; Larson 1977). Moreover, professional autonomy represents the outcome of competition and conflict between professional and managerial groups and not directly the outcome of class struggle at the workplace, an essential component of Friedman's original analysis (see, for example, Friedman 1977: 83).

Friedman's analysis can only be a starting point as it is not concerned directly with the question of professionalism or the role of the state within the public sector. Yet professionalism is not unaffected by the strategies of the state. Indeed, certain professions can be said to have been promoted by the capitalist state to meet its requirements of social reproduction. Examples here would include accountants (Johnson 1972, 1982) and engineers (Larson 1977). Doctors, however, have been able to define the collaboration between themselves and the state much more than most professions. This has had a great deal to do with the dependency of the state on the profession in the organization and control of health care delivery (see, for instance, Larson 1977). It is my argument that responsible autonomy has long been the preferred strategy of the British state towards the medical profession.

This, however, would not be an accurate way of describing the actual relationship. Instead, the medical profession has long persisted in pursuing strategies and tactics to prevent their corporate selves being fully incorporated into the state apparatus of health care. A central plank of this strategy has been the claim to clinical autonomy which has enabled doctors to dominate the organization and control of the health care labour process. This claim is authorized, as it were, by the process of licensure. Yet what exactly comprises clinical autonomy individual doctors seem unable to define, at least according to one recent survey (Harrison and Schulz 1989: 199). In sociological terms, clinical autonomy is, essentially, the indetermination component of an indetermination/technicity (I/T) ratio. It is defined by its lack of definition by the profession (Jamous and Peloille 1970: 112). One researcher who has attempted to identify the substantive nature of clinical autonomy is Tolliday (1978: 44). She identified four kinds of claims which have been made by doctors. These are:

- the right to independent practice;
- the right to refuse an individual patient;
- the responsibility to lead and coordinate other health professions;
- the over-arching primacy of medical knowledge.

These constitute an ideal-typical characterization of clinical autonomy. Individual doctors will be constrained according to their career status; junior doctors technically do not enjoy clinical autonomy but operate on behalf of the consultant who does. Similarly, the division of labour between consultants from different specialties working on a complex case (for example, a road accident victim with internal and head injuries) constrains the autonomy of individual doctors. Nevertheless, it is the doctors, and no one other group, who exercise clinical autonomy. This means of legitimating their ascendancy within the hospital division of labour has, in addition, had the consequence of giving doctors the power to commit resources – through their treatment plans – that has been a major problem for health service plans and the United Kingdom government at least since the 1960s (Klein 1989: 83).

It is the profession's ability to sustain the claim to the primacy of medical knowledge, however, that is fundamental. It is this that underpins what Freidson (1970) has conceptualized as professional dominance. This is a multi-faceted concept, the components of which were recently listed by Light and Levine (1988: 12–13) in the United States context as follows:

- autonomy over work;
- control over the work of others in one's domain;
- cultural beliefs and deference;
- institutional power.

The authors argue that in face of various and powerful political pressures on the profession over recent years (including pressures for cost-containment), the 'situation begs for a reformulation' (1988: 13). The profession's 'dominance' is seen as being institutionally rooted and vulnerable to encroachment, notably from the state. Any attempt, however, to incorporate the profession directly into the state apparatus has always been strongly resisted both in the United Kingdom and the United States, although the rhetoric of each has varied from one another. The United Kingdom profession has been less attached, for instance, to the fee-for-service principle so beloved of their American counterparts (Harrison and Schulz 1989).

The distinction between a state-defined responsible autonomy and an independent (that is, autonomous) status based on a claim to clinical autonomy (and maintained by an organized profession) might be said to be that between organizational and institutional control (Dent 1991). To explain, organizational control refers to the rules imposed by the state bureaucracy with the intent of limiting the profession's autonomy within the work situation. As Abercrombie and Urry say: 'Bureaucracy is . . . Janus-faced, for it is a system of constraint. Service-class workers benefit from bureaucratic employment in that they have relative autonomy, but they are also relatively constrained by bureaucratic rules' (1983: 121). Professionalization, by contrast, is characterized by an alternative, institutional, mode of control. This refers to the ability of an organized profession to define the extent of its members' autonomy within the work situation. It is important to note, however, that the distinction between organizational and institutional control is, in reality, far from clear-cut. Both types of control are tendencies rather than absolutes. The professional autonomy of doctors is some-thing that has been constantly negotiated and renegotiated between state and profession since the former has become directly involved in the delivery of health care. Initially, the predominant mode of professional autonomy resulted from the kind of state formations that emerged, first, during the nineteenth century when the modern form of the medical profession was established and, subsequently, with the establishment of the welfare state and the National Health Service (Johnson 1982: 189).

THE NATIONAL HEALTH SERVICE, HEALTH MAINTENANCE ORGANIZATIONS AND CLINICAL BUDGETING

The National Health Service has proven to be an essential part of the postwar consensus (Gough 1979) which any British government would need to be very wary of dismantling. But in establishing the system the state had provided the medical profession with an institutional power base that made it insensitive to demands to exercise a responsible autonomy. The profession has been able to enjoy the relatively unconstrained professional autonomy of the traditional intel-lectuals of Gramsci (1971) rather than being incorporated and restructured as organic 'intellectuals' (Abercrombie and Urry 1983: 147). This situation has been a major challenge to the British state over the decades since the inception of the National Health Service in major part because of the difficulties in controlling health care costs. By the 1980s the escalating costs of health care provision (Abel-Smith 1984) had reached such levels that the Conservative government believed itself impelled to find new ways of organizing the National

Health Service in order to contain them. Something like 80 per cent of overall health costs are generated by doctors' medical decisions (Schroeder 1980). It is unsurprising, therefore, that one of the principal strategies adopted by the government was to pressurize doctors to take on responsibility for cost-containment. But whereas previous attempts had been based on administrative reorganization plus exhortation, on this occasion the government was to attempt something far more radical – market competition.

The first move of the administration was the commissioning of the Griffiths Inquiry (Department of Health and Social Security 1983). Griffiths' recommend-ation was the replacement of consensus administration with more directive general management. This was very quickly accepted by the government (Ham 1985: 33–5). In this new scheme of things the general managers were 'charged with the responsibility for the efficient use of resources' (Elston 1991: 68), which meant, in practice, getting the doctors (as the biggest spenders) more centrally involved in decision-making processes within the hospitals. It is doubtful, however, that on its own the new system of general management was a serious challenge to the 'substance of consultant power across the NHS' (Cox 1991: 104). The strategy had been to entice doctors into general management as well as, more generally, educate doctors into understanding the imperatives of cost controls. In the event few doctors were enticed into becoming general managers (although by 1986 the figure had risen to 19 per cent [Cox 1991: 97]). But the intended aim of general management had been more fundamental – a direct challenge to the medical hegemony of doctors. This was an objective intended to be achieved with the aid of resource management and clinical budgeting (Thompson 1987; Scrivens 1988; Cox 1991: 103).

The Resource Management Initiative (Department of Health and Social Security 1986; Packwood *et al.* 1991) which followed shortly after the introduction of general management was designed to create a comprehensive system of man-agement budgeting as recommended by Griffiths (Department of Health and Social Security 1986: Appendix 1, para. 1). The term 'resource management' was adopted in order not to discourage medical (and nursing) involvement (Department of Health and Social Security 1986: 3, para. 5). The system of resource management was subsequently embodied in the White Paper *Working for Patients* (Department of Health 1989a: para. 2.15) enacted as the 1990 National Health Service and Community Care Act. Between the time of design-ing of the new resource management system and the government's White Paper *Working for Patients* the decision was taken to redesign the National Health Service according to the principles of the market. Initially, as Marmor and Plowden have recently explained, a 'purely Thatcherite model . . . would have been to turn [the National Health Service] . . . into a national insurance scheme, to get rid of as much state ownership of medical facilities as possible, and to encourage the purchase of private health insurance' (Marmor and Plowden 1991: 17). Politically, however, this strategy was impracticable and the government was forced to concede that in the United Kingdom access to medical care, free at the point of delivery, is a basic right of citizenship (Marmor and Plowden 1991;

Cox 1992: 34–8). Consequently, resource management and the National Health Service reorganization more generally (Department of Health 1989a) was a means less of privatizing the service than of introducing the competitive principles of the 'internal (quasi)-market' as an efficiency dynamic.

The inspirational model for the government was the Health Maintenance Organization, which can be briefly defined as follows: 'prepaid comprehensive capitation systems with financial incentives to maintain a subscriber's health by using no more services than are absolutely necessary' (Harrison and Schulz 1989: 208). Its injection into the National Health Service follows the advocacy of Alain Enthoven (1985) during the period of policy debate on the reorganization of the service in the mid-1980s (Klein 1989: 236; Marmor and Plowden 1991: 17).

This was not the only option that was looked at but it was the one in which the, now familiar, concept of an 'internal market' was advocated (Klein 1989: 236). As an idea it appeared to offer the prospect of containing costs by creating a competitive system within the National Health Service. In the words of the White Paper, *Working for Patients*, 'each District Health Authority's duty will be to buy the best service it can from its own hospitals, from other authorities' hospitals, from self-governing hospitals or from the private sector' (Department of Health 1989a: para. 4.13). Whilst 'hospitals, for their part, will have to satisfy Districts that they are delivering the best and most efficient service' (1989a: para. 4.13). In principle the National Health Service has now become analogous to a nationalized Health Maintenance Organization. Each District Health Authority now has to act as the 'Health Maintenance Organization' for its resident population with a duty to ensure the health services purchased are of a high quality and competitively priced. The new system was to be presented, by government, as a reorganization of the old National Health Service, not a rejection of its principles. The review concludes with the statement: 'The NHS is, and will continue to be, open to all, regardless of income, and financed mainly out of general taxation' (quoted in Klein 1989: 238). But while the system for the patient may remain, broadly, the same as it always has, the implications for the hospital doctors are very different. The new arrangements involve the doctors more directly in the management of hospitals than hitherto and, in the process, potentially subject their work to greater scrutiny. The traditional professional autonomy is beginning to give way to newer systems based on responsible autonomy. The organized medical profession, formally at least, accepts that medicine is delivered according to the priorities set by management as well as its own perceptions of the needs of the patients.

Having discussed these developments in terms of the strategies adopted by the state, I now turn to the question of the strategies adopted by the medical profession.

MEDICAL AUDIT, QUALITY ASSURANCE AND CLINICAL AUTONOMY

The strategy of the medical profession has tended to be one of prevarication. As is well known the profession is not a unitary one. Differences exist in the approaches adopted by the Royal Colleges and the British Medical Association as well as between the profession's leaders and the doctors at the 'grass roots'. Nevertheless, a general pattern is discernible and this is most apparent in relation to the issue of medical audit. This has been a leitmotiv of profession/state relations since the 1960s. This form of peer review, in its modern form, is premised on a systems model developed in the United States initially by Donabedian (1966). The model comprises three elements, structure, process and outcome which together define the components of medical audit within modern medicine (see Table 6.1).

The medical profession generally has preferred medical audit of the 'process' kind as it can remain directly under their control for only they can be the judge of a doctor's performance (Donabedian 1966: 168; Shaw 1980a: 1256–8). It is also the case that 'in practice, it is exceedingly difficult to derive feasible measures of outcome that can be actually used in evaluating the effectiveness and efficiency of services' (Butler and Vaile 1984: 127). This is because it is often difficult to (a) identify the precise outcome sought (for example, extend life or improve its quality); (b) establish the causal links between treatment and outcome; and (c) acquire the data.

Traditionally, British doctors have tended to treat medical audit with great circumspection. It originated in the United States with the establishment, by the American College of Surgeons, of the National Standardization Program for hospitals back in 1919.[2] Originally medical audits were little more than 'case meetings' or 'chart reviews' where the management of the patient was discussed. The surgical specialities would also hold mortality and morbidity meetings which some observers have argued function less as an audit and more as an opportunity to discuss 'interesting' cases or, where the death of a patient has occurred as a cathartic exercise (Arluke 1977; Millman 1977). In the process, however, they also function to socialize neophyte doctors and hence strengthen professional autonomy (Bosk 1979).

It was the introduction of the Medicare and Medicaid programmes in the United States in 1965 that, for the first time, meant public funds were to be used to reimburse physicians and hospitals for providing medical care to the aged and the poor (Freidson 1976: 288). The cost of these programmes was much higher than anticipated and led to the introduction of utilization reviews. These were designed to be checks on the economic (that is, financial) efficiency of the treatments given. But this form of audit proved to be too cumbersome and very

Table 6.1 The medical audit model

Structure	Process	Outcome
Hospital facilities and equipment, skill and qualification of staff	The clinic work processes directly the doctors' control	The patients' condition after treatment (i.e. morbidity, mortality and quality of life)

expensive (Freidson 1976; McSherry 1976). This led to a switch of emphasis from the evaluation of cost to one of quality of care as measured by medically defined criteria (Shaw 1980b). The responsible body involved was the Professional Standards Review Organization, which was established in 1972 (Sanazaro 1974; Brook and Avery 1976). Instead of reviewing individual cases, explicit, written, criteria for judging the adequacy of the care would be established beforehand (by the senior medical staff) for the medical audit committee. The medical records staff had the responsibility for monitoring the clinical records and when discrepancies were found would bring them to the attention of this committee (Sanazaro 1974; Shaw 1980b).

This change of emphasis from cost to quality was the result, at least in part, of the American Medical Association's strategy to avoid outside controls being applied to the profession (Westin 1976: 54; Krause 1977: 290–3). The profession was keen to defend the traditional (professional) autonomy against the demands for doctors to adopt a greater responsible autonomy. Even so, the implementation of federally mandated peer review met with considerable hostility from the membership (Krause 1977: 292; Björkman 1989: 55). A similar situation emerged in Britain and with similar consequences.

In the United Kingdom procedures have existed for the evaluation of health care. A good illustration of this is the Confidential Enquiry into Maternal Deaths (Godber 1976: 23–33; Butler and Vaile 1984: 168–9) which has been in existence since 1952. There is, also, the Confidential Enquiry into Perioperative Deaths, which is currently much cited as the example of 'good practice' (Department of Health, 1989b: 4). This is a major study of all deaths within thirty days of surgical operation. Another approach is that of the Oxford Medical Record Linkage system. This is a system of interlinking medical records at different hospitals designed to provide a comprehensive patient data-base (Henderson *et al.* 1989).

Pressure for doctors in the United Kingdom to adopt medical audit can be traced back to the introduction of the 'Cogwheel' reforms in the mid-1960s. Just as is the case now the Department of Health was committed to challenging the hospital doctors on the cost and effectiveness of medical work. There were two reports, one for England and Wales (Godber 1967) and the other for Scotland (Brotherstone 1967). Both reports recommended the introduction of a 'divisional system of staffing within NHS hospitals similar to that widely used in North America' (British Medical Journal 1967). It was only the Scottish report, however, that contained any specific reference to medical audit (Lancet 1967). Nevertheless, even the 'Cogwheel' report for England and Wales made specific reference to 'the review of clinical practice' (quoted in Forsyth 1967: 5). The British Medical Association and the Royal Colleges largely ignored the recommendations of 'Cogwheel' on this matter and the subject of medical audit did not emerge again as a major issue until 1971. This time the organized profession was concerned that the proposed National Health Service reorganization (Department of Health and Social Security 1972) would include a system of medical audit organized and controlled by the new specialism of community medicine. But, following lobbying from the British Medical Association, the profession was reassured by the Department of Health and Social Security that the new specialism of community medicine would not be used to operate as a system of clinical audit (British Medical Journal 1973: 29).

It was during this period leading up to the 1974 reorganization that the leadership at the British Medical Association began to recognize, as had the organized profession in the United States earlier, that medical audit had potential as a strategy to defend the professional autonomy of doctors. This strategy was first discussed in public on 20 November 1971 when the *British Medical Journal* published a lead article which directly linked the reorganization of the National Health Service with the issue of medical audit. The 'leader' was concerned with a book of essays, edited by McLachlan, entitled *Challenge for Change* (1971). The key point was that the author was recommending that the medical profession adopt a system, under its control, for 'the monitoring of the quality of health care' (British Medical Journal 1971: 443).

The strategy that the profession subsequently developed, however, was a flawed one. This was because the British Medical Association leadership was unable to convince its membership of the merits of the case. It took until 1981 before the policy of medical audit was finally accepted by the membership (British Medical Journal 1981). This seriously weakened the British Medical Association in its negotiations with government.

The organized profession's problems were further compounded by other related developments during the 1970s which threatened to mark the introduction of even more externally imposed controls – most notably, the establishment of the Hospital Advisory Service and the Health Commissioner or 'Ombudsman' (Klein 1989: 163–4). But it was the setting up of the Committee of Inquiry into the Regulation of the Medical Profession (Merrison 1975) that gave rise to particular concern at the time. Initially the profession was worried that the Committee might recommend a system of medical audit not fully under medical control. Towards the end of 1973, however, Dr Merrison came seeking advice from the British Medical Association on the question of 'competence to practise' (that is, medical audit). He accepted its suggestion that it would set up its own professional inquiry into the subject (British Medical Journal 1973).

The internal inquiry was chaired by E. A. J. Alment (Consultant Obstetrician and Gynaecologist). Its membership was drawn from the Royal Colleges and their Faculties as well as the British Medical Association (Alment 1976: 1). The Committee report can only be described as anodyne. On the specific issue of medical audit the Committee found 'peer-group reviews' and 'self-assessments' acceptable only as far as they were for educational purposes and involved no sanctions (Alment 1976: para. 9.12). Medical audit was viewed as 'threatening to a professional' on the grounds that the establishment of norms of good practice might be interpreted as rules for doctors to obey. Moreover, these norms might be used by 'employers and others to serve their own purposes' (Alment 1976: para. 6.9). Some five years later Alment confessed that the major reason for the cautious tone of the report resulted from the Committee's concern to avoid any polarization within the Committee or any antagonism within the wider profession (Alment 1981). The inadequacies of the Alment Committee's report seriously undermined the profession's ability to influence the subsequent Royal Commission (Merrison 1979). Moreover, the profession had great difficulty in 'cobbling together' a workable consensus in the period immediately prior to the publication of the Royal Commission on the National Health Service in 1979.

In its evidence to the Royal Commission the British Medical Association equivocated over the issue of medical audit, commenting that 'its place . . . in health care is still controversial', but it was to be inevitable that it should be carried out by the profession as a whole (British Medical Journal 1977: 301). The British Medical Association also regretted 'any suggestion that there should be "medical audit" by the state' (British Medical Journal 1977: 301). The Royal Commission was not impressed and in its Report commented, 'we are not convinced that the profession generally regards the introduction of audit or peer review . . . with a proper sense of urgency' (Merrison 1979: para. 12.56). It recommended that 'a planned programme for the introduction of audit or peer review . . . should be set up for the health professions by their professional bodies and progress monitored by the *health departments*' (Merrison 1979: para. 63; emphasis added). This is exactly what is contained in the current White Paper (Department of Health 1989a) and Working Paper 6 (Department of Health 1989b). Similarly, the 1979 Report, also favoured doctors becoming their own resource managers with their own budgets (Perrin 1979).

The 1979 Report contained the same general conclusions in regard to the medical profession as does the 1989 White Paper (Department of Health 1989a). But, in-between times, the now Conservative government worked assiduously during the 1980s to try to transform the culture of the National Health Service to facilitate these changes. The general strategy has been to encourage a number of doctors to take on a management role within the hospitals. This has been done by inviting selected hospital consultants to become 'clinical directors'. In this new role these doctors become directly responsible for the costs and quality of their specialty and (as part of the hospital management board) the hospital services generally (Mills 1989: 19).

THE INTERNAL MARKET AND QUALITY ASSURANCE

Turning now to the issue of the internal market, what the Department of Health and others that Klein (1989: 5) referred to collectively as the rationalist paternalists wanted was that hospital consultants become resource managers (see Merrison 1979). But it has been the market reformers, to adopt the term used by Alford (1972), who have seemingly brought about the changes necessary to get hospital consultants to take responsibility for their clinical budgets. As Griffiths commented: 'Doctors should be closely involved in local management through the development of management budgets for which they would be accountable' (Department of Health and Social Security 1983: 2). What is emerging is a revised version of the Health Maintenance Organization model in which the hospitals and their staff 'sell' (that is, contract) their services to the District Health Authority. The district management, for its part, is mandated to measure not only the cost of the service offered but also its quality (Department of Health 1989a: para. 2.11; Department of Health 1989b).

While medical audit refers to peer review, quality assurance concerns the quality of health care delivery more generally. Moreover, quality assurance involves all aspects of health care delivery, including nursing and paramedical services, as well as surveys of patients' levels of satisfaction with their treatment. This distinction, between peer review and quality assurance, however, is not one recognized within the White Paper, nor the relevant Working Paper (No. 6: Medical Audit). Instead, the two approaches are conflated into the following definition: '[The] systematic, critical analysis of the quality of medical care, including the procedures used for diagnosis and treatment, the use of resources, and the resulting outcome and quality of life for the patient' (Department of Health 1989b: para. 1.1). Nowhere here is the notion of successful surgery on a patient who, unfortunately, died, the common example given by doctors as a means of distinguishing the two practices. This new all-embracing concept of audit would force doctors, if it is fully implemented, to consider directly the costs of their clinical work and be more conscious of the 'outcomes' than has previously been the case.

Recent studies reported by Harrison and Schulz (1989: 203) reveal that doctors 'regard overall financial limitations as being legitimate restrictions on their autonomy . . . [but] did not see a legitimate role for peer review or quality assurance'. Under the requirements of the White Paper (Department of Health 1989a) however, medical audit and quality assurance are essential requirements of the new arrangements. Moreover, we find additional distinctions being made between medical and clinical audits – the difference being that the former only relates to the work of the clinicians while the latter concerns the whole health care team (including nurses, paramedics and so on) (Shaw and Costain 1989).

Currently, it is the explicit inclusion of 'outcome' measures that has become a central issue in the debate. In Working Paper 6 it is argued: '[There] is a need to develop a comprehensive set of measures of the outcome of much of the work of . . . doctors' (Department of Health 1989b: para. 2.3). Moreover, the Standing Medical Advisory Committee has been asked 'to consider how the quality of medical care can best be improved by means of medical audit, and *on the development of indicators of clinical outcome*' (para. 2.4.; emphasis added). It seems that the difficulties outlined earlier (Butler and Vaile 1984: 127–8) are no longer considered insurmountable by the policy advisers. Already work is being published on the use of 're-admission rates' as just such an indicator and one that is relatively uncomplicated to measure (Greener 1989: 12–13; Henderson *et al.* 1989: 709–13). This approach may be useful for acute cases, but in the area of chronic illness the 'outcome' is less certain, it being more a matter of the alleviation of suffering than the curing of the disease. Moreover, 're-admission rates' fail to identify patients' qualitative dissatisfactions with the outcome, which would, in any case, be difficult to measure (Cochrane 1971; Illsley 1980;

Butler and Vaile 1984). Nevertheless, the Royal Colleges now view 'outcome' as the most relevant indicator for medical audit purposes (see, for instance, Royal College of Physicians 1989: 2.4). Despite the formal commitment of the Royal Colleges to outcome measures, however, much emphasis remains on process audit, as the following quote, from the director of the medical audit programme at the King's Fund for Health Services Development, indicates:

> [Medical] audit relates to practices initiated directly by doctors. It . . . is primarily clinical . . . its focus is the *process and results* of medical care. . . . Medical audit is more systematic, quantified, and formal than traditional clinical ward rounds, meetings, and case presentations but shares with these the objectives of better patient care and education.
>
> (quoted in Shaw and Costain 1989: 498; emphasis added)

Note the difference of emphasis to the terms used in Working Paper 6 of the White Paper (Department of Health 1989b). There is no mention here of resources and the quality of life for patients is, at best, only hinted at. Improvement of quality, however, may not be the central rationale for the emphasis on auditing outcomes, for, as Enthoven pointed out, 'errors and complications are costly. Reviewing quality and taking corrective action . . . helps reduce costs' (1985: 44). Thus, it is hardly surprising that the government was to utilize the National Audit Office and the Public Accounts Committee as the means of assessing the general quality of care within the National Health Service (National Audit Office 1988; Public Accounts Commission 1989). The National Audit Office (1988: para. 1), in particular, was concerned from the outset to investigate the issue of medical audit in relation to the financial management of the National Health Service. In addition, the Public Accounts Commission (1989: para. 9) concluded that it might be necessary for audit to be covered through some form of contractual arrangement. District Health Authorities, in assessing which hospitals to contract with, will have to take the quality of care record – as well as price – into account. In this climate hospitals will have to decide whether to compete primarily on cost or a mix of cost and quality. Assuming, that is, that there is sufficient over-capacity within the system to facilitate market competition between hospitals.

With the mandated systems of quality control in place the patient as consumer, so the argument runs, need have no fear that market-led health care means a worsening service. There is, nevertheless, some evidence from the United States that clinical decisions are affected detrimentally by financial considerations within the Health Maintenance Organizations (see, for example, Hillman 1989: 86–92). Within the pages of the *British Medical Journal* Quam, in her critique of the White Paper proposals, has also argued forcibly against the introduction of the system in the United Kingdom on the grounds that, in the United States, 'burgeoning costs in the competitive system have coincided with persistent concerns over the quality of care . . . [and] low rates of patient satisfaction' (1989: 448). Whether the reorganization of the National Health Service leads to the improvement or decline in the quality of care, the changes do involve a fundamental change in the relationship between doctors and the state. Doctors have conceded that clinical autonomy is now to be subject to resource constraints. Moreover, it would appear from the research of Harrison and Schulz (1989: 203) mentioned earlier that generally they are not discontented by this erosion. In principle the new organizational arrangements involve the medical profession accepting the principles of responsible autonomy within an overall system of managerial control.

CONCLUSION

Hospital doctors in the United Kingdom have long enjoyed an extensive professional autonomy, one that has been premised on the state's dependency (see, for instance, Klein 1989). This dependency has been the consequence of the profession's own historically won ascendancy within the health care division of labour as much as it relates to its specific skills and knowledge. The nature of this dependency relationship now appears to be changing in some significant ways. Hospital doctors in the United Kingdom are finding themselves increasingly constrained by detailed rules concerning the quality and cost of their work. The profession has, finally, agreed to accept a more 'responsible autonomy' within the National Health Service and to cooperate with the introduction of resource management and new systems of quality control. Whether this new arrangement will become permanent rests more on the survival of the new organizational arrangements than on the profession's ability to recover some of its old syndicalist dominance.

While the government has been able to privatize virtually all of the nationalized industries and municipal services it has been unable to do the same with the National Health Service. Enthoven's intervention and advocacy of the Health Maintenance Organization model was therefore crucial in permitting the introduction of market principles within the National Health Service without privatization.

The state and the medical profession have been, more or less, continually in conflict over the issue of the resource/financial implications of clinical autonomy since, at least, the mid-1960s with the introduction of the 'Cogwheel' reforms. Negotiations, however, have always taken place within the framework of a centralized health service. Only by restructuring the health service and separating the allocative and operational decisions (Pahl and Winkler 1974: 114–15) has the administration been able to undermine the doctors' traditional dominance organizationally. As a consequence of the new arrangements doctors, in principle, no longer will have the ability to commit (allocate) additional resources as a consequence of their clinical decisions alone (see, for instance, Klein 1989: 83). Doctors will retain their control over the work situation (operational decisions), but allocative decisions will now become a managerial prerogative.

These fundamental changes in the National Health Service and profession/ state relations do not, however, constitute any 'proletarianization' of doctors. As McKinlay and Arches (1985) argue in the North American context, they still retain '*control over certain prerogatives relating to the location, content and essentiality of [their] task activities*' (quoted in Elston 1991; original emphasis).

This is so even if they perceive themselves as suffering a loss of occupational status as Larson (1980) and Derber (1983) have argued. Instead the doctors are undergoing an increase in the organizational control of the state (mediated by the internal market) at the expense of their own collective institutional control of the organized profession. This represents a change to what I have called responsible autonomy. This modification has not been at the expense of the doctors' dominant position within hospitals. But they have had to accept that they are no longer the only arbiters of health care delivery. With the establishment of resource management and the new producer–provider relations within the National Health Service, management now have the power to decide to which hospitals patients are to be referred. All this adds up to a radical readjustment rather than a class revolution.

The long-term strategy of the state administration in Britain has been to incorporate hospital consultants more fully within a system of organizational control. The earlier attempts to introduce a measure of cost-effectiveness into clinical care associated with the introduction of the divisional system of medical organization and the National Health Service reorganization of 1974 were unsuccessful because no way could be found comprehensively to breach the profession's resistance. It has only been with the adoption of the Thatcherite policies of replacing managerialism with (quasi)-market mechanisms that the profession's resistance to systematic clinical budgeting and medical audit has begun to be eroded. These changes, which are by no means complete or inevitable, have been brought about primarily as a consequence of economic pressure. It would seem that, in Alford's (1972) terms, the market reformers and not the bureaucratic rationalizers have won the day. It remains to be seen, however, whether the new management and quasi-market systems will actually work (see Packwood *et al.* 1991) or whether the doctors, or sufficient numbers of them, are any good at management.

NOTES

1 The contrast between organic and traditional professions derives from the discussion by Gramsci (1971) on intellectuals.
2 The roots of the National Standardization Program can be traced directly to the Flexner Report on medical education of 1910 (Roemer and Friedman 1971: 36–7). It is also important to note that the Program reflected the interests of the organized profession for it was, in practice, a response of the private interest of the doctors to the competitive anarchy of the market and one which enabled them to enhance their status and income levels (Maynard 1978: 7).

REFERENCES

Abel-Smith, B. (ed.) (1984) *Cost Containment in Health Care: A Study of 12 European Countries, 1977–83*, London: Bedford Square Press/NCCO.
Abercrombie, N. and Urry, J. (1983) *Capital, Labour and the Middle Classes*, Hemel Hempstead: Allen & Unwin.

Alford, R. R. (1972) 'The political economy of health care: dynamics without change', *Politics and Society* Winter: 127–64.

Alment, E. A. F. (1976) *Competence to Practise: The Report of a Committee of Enquiry Set Up for the Medical Profession in the UK*, London: HMSO.

—— (1981) 'Prologue: looking back on "competence to practise"', in G. McLachlan (ed.), *Reviewing Practice in Medical Care*, London: NPHT.

Arluke, A. (1977) 'Social control rituals in medicine', in R. Dingwall, C. Heath, M. Reid and M. Stacey (eds), *Health Care and Health Knowledge*, London: Croom Helm.

Björkman, J. W. (1989) 'Politicizing medicine and medicalizing politics: physician power in the United States', in G. Freddi and J. W. Björkman (eds), *Controlling Medical Professionals: The Comparative Politics of Health Governance*, London: Sage.

Bosk, C. L. (1979) *Forgive and Remember: Managing Medical Failure*, London: University of Chicago Press.

Braverman, H. (1974) *Labor and Monopoly Capital*, New York: Monthly Review Press.

British Medical Journal (1967), 'Modernizing hospital medicine', *British Medical Journal* 4 November: 252–3.

—— (1971) 'Challenge to change', *British Medical Journal* 20 November: 443.

—— (1973) 'NHS reorganization: BMA letter to profession: progress report', *British Medical Journal* Supplement, 3 February: 29–30.

—— (1977) 'Submission of evidence' *British Medical Journal* 29 January: 301–3.

—— (1981), 'From the ARM: medical audit', *British Medical Journal* Supplement, 18 July: 243–4.

Brook, R. H. and Avery, A. D. (1976) 'Quality assurance mechanisms in the United States: from there to where?', in G. McLachlan (ed.), *A Question of Quality?*, London: NPHT/Oxford University Press.

Brotherstone, J. H. F. (1967) *Organisation of Medical Work in the Hospital Services in Scotland*, Edinburgh: HMSO.

Butler, J. R. and Vaile, M. S. B. (1984) *Health and Health Services*, London: Routledge & Kegan Paul.

Cochrane, A. (1971) *Effectiveness and Efficiency*, London: NPHT.

Cox, D. (1991) 'Health service management – a sociological view: Griffiths and the non-negotiated order of the hospital', in J. Gabe, M. Calnan and M. Bury (eds), *The Sociology of the Health Service*, London: Routledge.

—— (1992) 'Crisis and opportunity in health service management', in R. Loveridge and K. Starkey (eds), *Continuity and Crisis in the NHS*, Buckingham: Open University Press.

Dent, M. (1991) 'Autonomy and the medical profession: medical audit and management control', in C. Smith, D. Knights and H. Wilmott (eds), *White-Collar Work: The Non-Manual Labour Process*, London: Macmillan.

Department of Health (1989a) *Working for Patients*, London: HMSO.

—— (1989b) *Medical Audit, NHS Review*, Working Paper 6, London: HMSO.

Department of Health and Social Security (1972) *Management Arrangements for the Reorganised National Health Service*, London: HMSO.

—— (1983) *National Health Service Management Inquiry*, London: HMSO.

—— (1986) *Health Services Management: Resource Management (Management Budgeting) in Health Authorities*, Circular HN (86) 34, November.

Derber, C. (1983) 'Sponsorship and the control of physicians', *Theory and Society* 12(5): 561–601.

Donabedian, A. (1966) 'Evaluating the quality of medical care', *Milbank Quarterly* 64(3), Part 2: 166–206.

Elston, M. A. (1991) 'The politics of professional power: medicine in a changing health service', in J. Gabe, M. Calnan and M. Bury (eds), *The Sociology of the Health Service*, London: Routledge.

Enthoven, A. C. (1985) *Reflections on the Management of the National Health Service*, London: NPHT.

Forsyth, G. (1967) *In Low Gear?* London: NPHT.

Freddi, G. (1989) 'Problems of organizational rationality in health systems: political controls and policy options', in G. Freddi and J. W. Björkman (eds), *Controlling Medical Professionals: The Comparative Politics of Health Governance*, London: Sage.

Freidson, E. (1970) *Professional Dominance: The Social Structure of Medical Care*, New York: Atherton.

—— (1976) 'The development of administration accountability in health services', *American Behavioral Scientist* 19(3): 286–98.

Friedman, A. L. (1977) *Industry and Labour*, London: Macmillan.

Godber, G. (1967) *First Report of the Joint Working Party on the Organization of Medical Work in Hospitals*, London: HMSO.

—— (1976) 'The Confidential Enquiry into Maternal Deaths', in G. McLachlan (ed.), *A Question of Quality?*, London: NPHT/Oxford University Press.

Gough, I. (1979) *The Political Economy of the Welfare State*, London: Macmillan.

Gramsci, A. (1971) *Selections From the Prison Notebooks of Antonio Gramsci*, eds Q. Hoare and G. N. Smith, London: Lawrence & Wishart.

Greener, B. (1989) 'Re-admission rates: an indicator of the quality of care', *British Journal of Health Care Computing* 6(10): 12–13.

Ham, C. (1985) *Health Policy in Britain*, 2nd edition, Basingstoke: Macmillan.

Harrison, S. and Schulz, R. I. (1989) 'Clinical autonomy in the UK and the USA: contrasts and convergence', in G. Freddi and J. W. Björkman (eds), *Controlling Medical Professionals: The Comparative Politics of Health Governance*, London: Sage.

Henderson, J., Goldacre, M. J., Graveney, M. J. and Simmons, H. M. (1989) 'Use of medical record linkage to study readmission rates', *British Medical Journal* 16 September: 709–13.

Hillman, A. L. (1989) 'How do financial incentives affect physicians? Clinical decisions and the financial performance of HMOs', *New England Journal of Medicine* 13 July: 81–2.

Illsley, R. (1980) *Professional or Public Health?*, London: NPHT.

Jamous, H. and Peloille, B. (1970) 'Professions or self-perpetuating systems? Changes in the French university-hospital system', in J. A. Jackson (ed.), *Professions and Professionalization*, Cambridge: Cambridge University Press.

Johnson, T. J. (1972) *Professions and Power*, London: Macmillan.

—— (1982) 'The state and the professions: peculiarities of the British', in A. Giddens and G. Mackenzie (eds), *Social Class and the Division of Labour: Essays in Honour of Ilya Neustadt*, Cambridge: Cambridge University Press.

Klein, R. (1989) *The Politics of the National Health Service*, 2nd edition, London: Longman.

Krause, E. (1977) *Power and Illness*, New York: Elsevier.

Lancet (1967) 'Chairman elect', *Lancet* 11 November: 1027–8.

Larson, M. S. (1977) *The Rise of Professionalism: A Sociological Analysis*, London: University of California Press.

—— (1980) 'Proletarianization and educated labor', *Theory and Society* 9(1): 131–75.

Light, D. W. and Levine, S. (1988) 'The changing character of the medical profession: a theoretical overview', *The Milbank Quarterly* 66 (Suppl. 2): 10–32.

McKinlay, J. B. and Arches, J. (1985) 'Towards the proletarianization of physicians', *International Journal of Health Services* 15: 161–95.

McLachlan, G. (ed.) (1971) *Challenge for Change*, London: NPHT.

McSherry, C. K. (1976) 'Quality assurance', *Surgery* 80(1): 122–9.

Marmor, T. R. and Plowden, W. (1991) 'Spreading the sickness', *Times Higher Educational Supplement* 25 October: 17.

Maynard, A. (1978) 'The medical profession and the efficiency and equity of health services', *Social and Economic Administration* 12(1): 3–19.

Merrison, A. W. (1975) *Report on the Committee of Inquiry into the Regulation of the Medical Profession*, London: HMSO.
—— (1979) *Royal Commission on the National Health Service*, London: HMSO.
Millman M (1977) *The Unkindest Cut*, New York: Morrow & Co.
Mills, A. (1989) *Resource Management Initiative: Information Package – Acute Hospitals*, NHS RM Directorate, March.
National Audit Office (1988) *Quality of Clinical Care in NHS Hospitals*, London: HMSO.
Packwood, T., Keen, J. and Buxton, M. (1991) *Hospitals in Transition: The Resource Management Initiative*, Milton Keynes: Open University Press.
Pahl, R. E. and Winkler, J. T. (1974) 'The economic élite: theory and practice', in P. Stanworth and A. Giddens (eds), *Élites and Power in British Society*, Cambridge: Cambridge University Press.
Perrin, J. (1979) *Management of Financial Resources in the NHS*, Royal Commission on the NHS Research Paper 2, London: HMSO.
Public Accounts Commission (1989) *Quality of Clinical Care in NHS Hospitals*, London: HMSO.
Quam, L. (1989) 'Improving clinical effectiveness in the NHS: an alternative to the White Paper', *British Medical Journal* 12 August: 448–50.
Roemer, M. I. and Friedman, J. W. (1971) *Doctors in Hospitals*, Baltimore: Johns Hopkins University Press.
Royal College of Physicians (1989) *Medical Audit: A First Report. What, Why and How?*, London: Royal College of Physicians of London.
Sanazaro, P. J. (1974) 'Medical audit: experience in the USA', *British Medical Journal* 16 February: 271–4.
Schroeder, S. A. (1980) 'Variations in physician practice patterns: a review of medical cost implications', in E. J. Carels, D. Neuhauser and W. B. Stason (eds), *The Physician and Cost Control*, Cambridge, Mass.: Oelschlager, Gunn & Hain.
Scrivens, E. (1988) 'The management of clinicians in the National Health Service', *Social Policy and Administration* 22(1): 22–34.
Shaw, C. D. (1980a) 'Aspects of audit: 1. The background', *British Medical Journal* 24 May: 1256–7.
—— (1980b) 'Aspects of audit: 5. Looking forward to audit', *British Medical Journal* 21 June: 1509–11.
Shaw, C. D. and Costain, D. W. (1989) 'Guide-lines for medical audit: seven principles', *British Medical Journal* 19 August: 498–9.
Thompson, D. (1987) 'Coalitions and conflict in the National Health Service: some implications for general management', *Sociology of Health and Illness* 9(2): 127–53.
Tolliday, H. (1978) 'Clinical autonomy', in E. Jacques (ed.), *Health Services*, London: Heinemann.
Westin, A. F. (1976) *Computers, Health Records and Citizen Rights*, Washington, DC: National Bureau of Standards, Monograph No. 157, US Printing Office.

7 The changing response of the medical profession to alternative medicine in Britain
A case of altruism or self-interest?

Mike Saks

Any rounded consideration of health professions in Britain should include not only their operation within orthodox boundaries, but also the interface between orthodox and unorthodox medicine. This is underlined by the rapid growth in popularity of alternative medicine in this country in modern times, following a similar pattern to that of many other parts of Europe (Sharma 1992). This interest has covered a wide range of therapies – from chiropractic and healing at one end of the spectrum to reflexology and aromatherapy at the other – that still lie outside mainstream medicine in terms of the level of official acknowledgement and support (Saks 1992a). With spiralling public interest in such therapies over the past two or three decades variously related to such factors as the perceived crisis of orthodox medicine and a desire for greater personal engagement in health care (Saks 1994), the future relationship between the medical profession and alternative medicine in Britain has become a significant matter of public debate. This debate partly centres on the role of the state, especially in view of the passage of the 1993 Osteopaths Act, which – in providing for the protection of title of qualified osteopathic practitioners within a legislatively underwritten framework of self-regulation (Standen 1993) – has created a climate of heightened expectation amongst practitioners of alternative therapies about their prospects which may or may not be realized in the future.

This chapter discusses the changing response of the medical profession to alternative medicine in Britain with particular reference to a case study of the recent medical reception of acupuncture, one of the more heavily utilized alternative therapies in this country (Fulder 1988). This exploration – which is undertaken in the broader context of the relationship between the professions, the public interest and the state – focuses on the extent to which this response represents that of a profession in transition from a narrowly self-interested stance to one that embodies a greater sense of public responsibility. The interpretation made of the part played by the medical profession in this field clearly has potential implications for future patterns of regulation by the state given its critical role in underwriting the privileged position of professions, not least in the health arena in Britain (Moran and Wood 1993). Here the medical profession enjoys, amongst other things, a legally enshrined monopoly in the state-financed National Health Service in contrast to non-medically qualified alternative practititioners who are predominantly focused in the private sector (Saks 1991a). However, before the reception that the medical profession has given to alternative medicine in general and acupuncture in particular in the contemporary era is considered, the long-standing sociological debate over the altruism of professional groups must first be outlined.

PROFESSIONAL ALTRUISM, SOCIOLOGY AND SOCIAL CHANGE

In this respect, the work of sociologists of the professions in the Anglo-American context on the pivotal question of how far professional groups subordinate their own interests to those of the wider society is sharply divided: up until the late 1960s the trait and functionalist literature on this subject generally held that professions lived up to their altruistic ideologies and were more oriented to the public good than parochial group interests; thereafter, sociologists working within the now dominant neo-Weberian and Marxist perspectives have tended to counter this stance with a more sceptical interpretation of the relationship between professional self-interests and the public interest. One problem with this chrono-logically polarized literature is that contributors from both camps have all too often derived their interpretations from predetermined positions as to whether professions place their own interests above those of the wider community, without basing their conclusions on rigorous analysis within a clearly defined theoretical and methodological framework capable of generating counterfactual conditions (Saks 1990). In consequence, the interpretation of the altruism claims of professions has hitherto largely been locked in a theoretical straitjacket in which it has been difficult or even impossible to conceptualize and examine possible changes in professional behaviour in this field.

Such deficiencies – which inhibit the systematic consideration of any trans-itional shifts in the orientations of professions in this area – are mirrored in work by sociologists in Britain and the United States on the medical profession on which this chapter focuses. This is illustrated by the frequently entrenched position adopted by the new orthodoxy which emerged in the 1970s and 1980s on the links between the ideology and reality of the professional altruism ideal in medicine (see, for example, Robson 1973; Esland 1980; and Navarro 1986); contributions within its compass have typically been critical of the balance struck by the medical profession between professional self-interests and the public interest, despite the early optimism of authors such as Marshall (1963) that doctors and other professional groups would meet their public responsibilities as defined by their professional codes as state intervention increased in Britain.

Crompton (1990) has suggested, however, that the critical portrayal of the medical profession in recent sociological literature has been tempered over the last few years by the beginnings of a reappraisal of its role in the British context. She argues that a more sympathetic view of the medical profession is emerging, largely because of the stand taken by doctors since the late 1980s as defenders of the National Health Service in face of attacks by the state on the principles of public provision in health care and the introduction of the internal market based on the White Paper, *Working for Patients* (Department of Health 1989). This image of a profession setting aside its own interests in favour of a broader concern with patient care throws into focus the significance of the question of how far the professions in general and the medical profession in particular change their approach to specific issue areas over time on the continuum from unenlightened self-interest to a more public-spirited frame of reference.

If lessons are to be learned from past work in the sociology of professions and this question is to be constructively addressed, an appropriate theoretical and methodological framework is needed for analysing at a collective level the activities of doctors and other professional occupations, which avoids making prior judgements about the fulfilment or otherwise of the altruism ideal. The two key constituents of such a framework are the construction of an operational concept of professional self-interests to weigh against other potential explanatory factors in specific decision-making situations, and the adoption of a viable notion of the public good, in relation to which the compatibility of the decisions taken by professional groups can reasonably be gauged (Saks 1990).

Developing this framework is a difficult task, even at the basic definitional level, not least because the concepts of the public interest and professional self-interest have been interpreted in so many diverse and contradictory ways from a range of perspectives in the social sciences. The strengths and weaknesses of these interpretations in appraising the altruism of the professions have been examined at length by the author elsewhere (see Saks 1985). As a result of this exercise and the author's own theoretical predilections, the notion of professional self-interests will be operationalized by basing judgements about their direction on an assessment of the achievement of benefits and the avoidance of costs in particular situations, largely with reference to wealth, power and prestige. Similarly, a relativistic concept of the public interest will be adopted, such that professional altruism claims are evaluated against the basic values of the society under scrutiny at the time of study. In Britain such judgements would be made against the the complex of social principles underpinning the British liberal-democratic state at a specific point in time – with particular consideration being given to the balance struck between the principles of seeking justice, promoting the general welfare, and securing the maximum amount of freedom compatible with these ends (Saks 1990).

Having established the rudiments of an analytical framework, the question of whether there has been any recent transitional movement in the balance between self-interests and wider social responsibilities manifested in the response of the British medical profession to alternative medicine can now be examined through the case study of acupuncture. Importantly, this case seems to follow a similar pattern to that of the medical reception of a number of other alternative therapies, not least because medical interest in this technique has increased in recent years as its popularity has grown (Saks 1994). Before moving on specifically to interpret the medical response to acupuncture from the viewpoint of the altruism debate in the changing context of modern Britain, the main dimensions of the medical response to this procedure need to be briefly elaborated in the period from the early 1960s to the present day.

THE RECENT RESPONSE OF THE MEDICAL PROFESSION TO ACUPUNCTURE

In presenting a thumbnail sketch of recent trends in the medical response to acupuncture, it should be stressed that this broad-ranging therapeutic modality based on the insertion of needles into the body is not a new phenomenon as far as Britain is concerned. As with such currently defined alternative therapies as herbalism and naturopathy, there have been flurries of medical interest in this subject in the past (see, for instance, Bynum and Porter 1987). The most significant of these in relation to acupuncture was in the early to mid-nineteenth century, after which this technique was marginalized until its revival in the 1950s and 1960s in this country (Saks 1985). In the period that followed, the response of the medical profession to this method seemed to pass through a significant watershed in the mid-1970s, which provides a helpful analytical division in outlining the general shape of the medical response to acupuncture in the thirty-year time span under consideration.

In the 1960s and first half of the 1970s it was evident that acupuncture continued to be generally rejected by the medical profession, following its resurrection in this country at the beginning of this period. In common with other areas of unorthodoxy, the very few medical practitioners of this ancient practice were stigmatized and shunned by their colleagues at this time, whilst the slowly expanding ranks of non-medical practitioners of this therapy were subjected to even greater hostility from within orthodox professional boundaries, not least from their medically qualified counterparts (Saks 1992b). Research into acupuncture and the teaching of it were also not officially sponsored and this subject received only the most peripheral attention in mainstream professional journals (Saks 1991b). This negative reception was exemplified by the incredulous medical response that was initially given to the media publicity showered upon the application of 'acupuncture anaesthesia' in major operations in China in the early 1970s – which was dismissively regarded as explicable in terms of socio-psychological factors such as hypnosis and the placebo reaction, rather than any real physical effect in its own right (Webster 1979). This was the low point from which acupuncture was to recover.

From the mid-1970s onwards the position changed substantially, to some extent mirroring that for alternative therapies more generally. Doctors and other health personnel within the orthodox division of labour increasingly took up the practice of acupuncture, such that there are probably now some 1,500 medical practitioners of the method in Britain (Saks 1992b). To these practitioners, moreover, should be added the high proportion of doctors who currently believe that acupuncture is a useful therapy (see, for example, Reilly 1983; Wharton and Lewith 1986) and the significant number of medical practitioners who are prepared to refer patients to its exponents (see, for instance, Nicholls and Luton 1986). This shift in interest has also been paralleled by a limited degree of support for acupuncture research from medically dominated funding bodies in institutions including St Bartholemew's Hospital and the Royal Edinburgh Hospital (Saks 1985), as well as the growing willingness of mainstream medical journals to publish material on acupuncture – which is exemplified by the fifty-seven published items on this subject in the *Lancet* and the *British Medical Journal* alone in the 1980s as compared with only two in the 1960s (Saks 1991b).

This apparent volte-face needs exploring to assess its compatibility with the view that there has been a shift in the philosophy of the medical profession from a narrow self-interested stance to one which more fully reflects the public responsibility of the profession within the British liberal-democratic state. This can be more fully explored in two stages: first, by considering the evidence for the link between the position of the medical profession on acupuncture and the dual concepts of professional self-interests and the public interest in the period up to the mid-1970s; and then by repeating the exercise in scrutinizing the changing response of the medical profession to acupuncture in the ensuing period up to the present day.

THE PERIOD FROM THE 1960s TO THE MID-1970s: THE PREVALENCE OF UNENLIGHTENED MEDICAL SELF-INTERESTS?

In looking at the evidence covering the first of these periods, it is quite clear that it was in the self-interests of the medical profession, as previously defined, to respond negatively to this therapeutic technique in the 1960s and early 1970s – both as regards the interests of the profession as a whole in relation to the relatively small group of lay practitioners of acupuncture and the specific interests of the medical élite, encompassing leading figures in the Royal Colleges and the British Medical Association, in relation to the even less numerous group of medical acupuncturists. The rejection of acupuncture – and most other forms of alternative medicine – at this time by the profession in general assuredly enabled this body to achieve benefits and minimize costs. In the specific case of acupuncture this was mainly because of the threat to the status and power of modern medicine posed by the traditional Yin–Yang theories adopted by most of the lay exponents of the method which were at variance with orthodox biomedicine and by the financial challenge to doctors that such independent practitioners were gradually beginning to mount in private practice across a broad range of conditions. Similarly, the interests of the medical élite lay in marginalizing medical acupuncturists – who were primarily drawn from the lower-status ranks of general practitioners – since their traditionally based practice at this time could readily have further augmented the external challenge to medical orthodoxy (Saks 1992b).

Such professional self-interests, moreover, seem to have been at the heart of the rejection of acupuncture at this time since the main alternative explanations of the rejection do not stand up at all well. This certainly applies to possible medical ignorance of the modality. The profession could not have failed to have been aware of acupuncture at this time given its long history in this country going back several centuries (Lu Gwei-Djen and Needham 1980) and its high profile in the media, culminating in the massive press attention given to the Chinese use of the technique in the early 1970s (Webster 1979). Such was the importance of the claims being made on behalf of acupuncture in a wide range of complaints, including pain and various chronic disorders from arthritis to asthma, that the method could scarcely have been rejected by the profession on the grounds of its lack of potential, particularly in light of the fact that it seemed to fill several notable gaps in the orthodox medical repertoire (Mann 1973). And while there were rare incidents at this time of collapsed lungs and haemorrhage linked to acupuncture treatment which raised issues about the safety of the technique (Macdonald 1982), these were not sufficient to have been overriding factors in any rejection, especially in view of the vulnerability of orthodox medicine itself in this period in the wake of the thalidomide disaster (Gould 1985). Cost could also barely have entered the equation given the cheapness of basic acupuncture equipment in an era marked by such expensive innovations as high-technology mass hospital births and coronary care units (Richman 1987). Nor indeed should the incompatibility of the more holistic traditional philosophy underpinning acupuncture with orthodox biomedicine have been a spur to its rejection, given the availability of Western theories of its operation like the 'gate-control' theory of Melzack and Wall (Lewith 1985) and the example set by the classical con-temporary practice of acupuncture alongside Western medicine in China (Shao 1988).

The notion that professional self-interests were a central part of the explan-ation of the rejection of acupuncture in the period up to the mid-1970s is also supported by the fact that the huge multi-national drug and medical equipment corporations do not seem to have directly influenced the proceedings; the out-come arrived at appears to have owed most to the long-established medical domination of decision-making, which gave force to the professional self-interests involved (Saks 1992b). As such, the medical profession seems to have trodden a similar path to that outlined by Larkin (1983) in relation to the professions supplementary to medicine in self-interestedly using its monopolistic position to defend its occupational territory. The evidence for the mainstream involvement of professional self-interests in the rejection of acupuncture by the medical profession in the 1960s and early 1970s does not necessarily imply, however, that this stance militated against the public interest, for the concepts of professional self-interest and the public interest are not necessarily incompatible (Saks 1985).

None the less, enough has so far been said to indicate that in this case the self-interested rejection of acupuncture by the medical establishment was not liable to have advanced the public good, as delineated in this chapter. Crucially, acupuncture – like a number of other alternative therapies at this time – appeared to have several significant potential advantages in comparison to existing bio-medical provision, including low cost, relative safety and enhanced therapeutic applicability in some areas (Saks 1992b). Yet in blocking its development both internally and externally the profession could be seen to have limited public access to this method and to have prejudiced the general welfare. Of course, lay acupuncturists were free to practise in the private sector under the common law, but were crucially disadvantaged by being excluded from the National Health Service (Inglis 1980). This meant that only orthodox health personnel were formally able to offer acupuncture treatment at no direct charge at the point of delivery in the state sector, with all its restrictive implications for freedom of choice. These restrictions were exacerbated by the inevitable geographical ine-qualities in access to the few medical and non-medical acupuncturists who were in existence in Britain at this time (Saks 1985).

This analysis, then, appears to bear out the view that the period from the 1960s to the mid-1970s was indeed marked by the effects of professional self-interests, which operated to the detriment of the wider society as far as acupuncture was concerned. This latter assessment is reinforced by the fact that the 1960s and early 1970s was an era in which greater political emphasis than today in the British liberal-democratic state was placed on advancing social justice (Dearlove and Saunders 1984), the cause of which the profession manifestly did not progress in this area. Irrespective, therefore, of whether doctors or non-medically qualified practitioners were best placed to deliver acupuncture treatment at this time – about which there might legitimately be debate in light of the variable standard of training in this practice both inside and outside of the profession – the stance of the medical profession did not seem to accord with the public interest, as defined in this chapter. But if unenlightened professional self-interests formed the main underpinning for the medical rejection of acupuncture in this period, what of the time span from the mid-1970s to the present day when the medical pendulum, as has been seen, swung a considerable distance in the direction of acupuncture?

THE PERIOD FROM THE MID-1970s TO THE PRESENT DAY: THE PREVALENCE OF PROFESSIONAL ALTRUISM?

At first sight it seems that only one conclusion can be reached as far as acu-puncture is concerned in this period – namely, that the medical profession did indeed altruistically subordinate its interests to the wider public good in relation to acupuncture, as its response was transformed from almost total rejection to a degree of acceptance following the mid-1970s. This interpretation, though, requires particularly close scrutiny.

Taking the relationship of the stance of the medical profession to the public interest first, it is true, as has been seen, that the profession moved to incorporate acupuncture into medicine after the mid-1970s, with all the associated increase in medical practice, research and publications in this area. However, the foothold that acupuncture obtained within medical orthodoxy – following that of such alternative therapies as homoeopathy (Nicholls 1988) – was sufficiently tenuous to challenge the public interest orientation of the profession. Certainly, the proportion of doctors practising acupuncture has remained comparatively small despite the growth of medical interest in the technique; acupuncture is also now primarily employed by doctors only in a very limited range of applications, the most predominant of which is pain; it is still not formally part of the orthodox medical school curriculum; and publicly and privately funded research into acupuncture by medically dominated bodies has yet to gain more than minimal support compared with other, more orthodox therapies (Saks 1992b).

These features hardly suggest a profession acting vigorously in the public interest, particularly in relation to the advancement of the general welfare in a situation in which greater evidence has now accumulated on the advantages of acupuncture – at least part of which is based on the randomized controlled trial methodology favoured by the profession – as the costs and limitations of ortho-dox medicine become even more apparent (Saks 1985). Nor does the limited response of the medical profession fit in with recent opinion poll data which have shown that a substantial majority of the British population want acupuncture and other more established forms of alternative medicine to be more widely available on the National Health Service (Saks 1991a). In this respect, whilst more doctors and allied health professionals are now practising acupuncture within the state sector, this is not keeping pace with the fast-growing public demand for this therapy (Fulder 1988), especially given its generally more restricted scope of application in the hands of medical practitioners. The altruistic credentials of the profession can therefore again be questioned in Britain in which increased political importance is now attached to the consumer in health provision (as highlighted by *The Patient's Charter* [Department of Health 1991]), but in which accessibility and freedom of choice in relation to acupuncture are limited – not least for those who cannot afford to purchase health care in the private sector.

A rather different interpretation of the position of the medical profession might have been justified had it made more strenuous efforts to facilitate the broader delivery of acupuncture through the expanding numbers of lay acu-puncturists in professionally organized groups – who now generally have a much sounder educational base and are more strongly focused around distinct codes of practice than in the period before the mid-1970s (Fulder 1988). In fact the reverse has occurred. While the amount of cooperation between doctors and lay acupunc-turists at grassroots level seems to have gradually increased, it has still been less common for doctors to refer patients to non-medical, as opposed to medical, exponents of acupuncture (see, for instance, Reilly 1983; Nicholls and Luton 1986), despite the fact that the former practitioners typically have a much longer training in this form of alternative therapy. At an institutional level, too, the medical profession has, if anything, intensified its attack on the characteristically wider-ranging classical practice of lay acupuncturists by emphasizing that it is unscientific and unsafe (Saks 1991b). Meanwhile active efforts have been made by the British Medical Acupuncture Society to exclude non-medically qualified exponents of acupuncture from the National Health Service (Saks 1992b). Needless to say, these actions have not helped to improve social class and geographical inequalities in access to this therapy.

This raises the question of why the medical professsion did not pursue its public obligations to acupuncture further in Britain in the period from the mid-1970s onwards. In light of the foregoing, the notion that the profession only took up acupuncture in a limited manner to protect the public from the quackery of unorthodox practitioners is not very persuasive. Nor can an adequate explanation easily be found in the comparative merits of biomedicine as regards acupuncture, given the shortcomings of medical orthodoxy relative to the strengths of acupuncture. And explanations centred on such factors as medical ignorance of the technique and the holistic basis of the therapy have become even less convincing in the period following the mid-1970s with the much heightened exposure of acupuncture in medical journals (Saks 1991b) and a growing commitment by some medical practitioners to facilitating interventions which see the patient as mind, body and spirit within orthodox medicine itself (Sharma 1992).

Since the medical profession again seems to have been the key body involved in restricting the availability of acupuncture, it is increasingly clear that far from professional self-interests being sacrificed in this area, they may actually have been the central factor underlying the state of affairs that developed from the mid-1970s to the present day. In terms of the balance of costs and benefits, it is easy to understand why the maintenance of hostility towards lay acupuncturists should have been in the self-interests of the profession in this period. It is important to note in this respect that the holistic philosophical tenets of much lay acupuncture continued to clash with the main therapeutic principles on which the power, status and financial security of most practitioners of biomedicine were based; that lay acupuncturists were not formally seeking any accommodation with orthodox medicine that involved taking on a subordinate status in the health care division of labour; and that acupuncture was one of the fastest expanding therapies in the field of unorthodox health care (Fulder 1988).

Although the fast-rising numbers of non-medically qualified acupuncturists were able more extensively to relieve the pressure on doctors in dealing with difficult patients with intractable conditions, their very expansion – together with the unification of the major non-medical acupuncture organizations under the umbrella of the Council for Acupuncture – enhanced the threat that they posed to the profession (Saks 1992b). This is especially apparent in the context of the rapid parallel growth that occurred amongst other alternative practitioners in Britain, which brought their overall numbers up to tens of thousands, and the increasing political support that was given to alternative medicine – most notably from the recently re-formed all-party Parliamentary Group on Alternative and Complementary Medicine (Saks 1991a). In this light, the interests of the medical profession were almost certainly institutionally best served by continuing to hold lay acupuncturists at a distance for fear that competition with unorthodox therapists might escalate across the board, in both the public and private sector.

Ironically, these same self-interests can also be seen to have primarily accounted for the few positive steps that the medical profession in Britain has made in relation to acupuncture since the mid-1970s. The limited encouragement given to medical acupuncturists within the profession marked a departure from previous policy, but served as a buffer against the developing challenge from without, in face of rapidly expanding public demand. Whilst there was a risk that this would further fan the flames of alternative practice in general, this was countered by channelling the practice of acupuncture within the profession to restricted areas such as pain and addictions through strategic control by the medical élite over career, publication and research opportunities (Saks 1985). This strategy was underwritten by legitimating neurophysiological explanations of the *modus operandi* of acupuncture linked to its analgesic effects, the most popular of which is now centred on the release of endorphins (Saks 1992b). These accounts also functioned to perpetuate the elevated position of the medical élite against the claims of insiders by emphasizing the orthodox knowledge base underpinning this therapy. The net result has in fact been to increase the scope for exploitation of acupuncture by doctors, whilst at the same time limiting public access to the more traditional wider-ranging forms of this therapy to the seeming detriment of the public interest.

THE MEDICAL PROFESSION, ALTRUISM AND ALTERNATIVE MEDICINE

But if the apparent change of position by the medical profession on acupuncture from unenlightened self-interests to a more altruistic approach in modern Britain is a chimera, this should not be too surprising given the tensions that have existed between the orthodox medical profession and alternative medicine since the state underwriting of medical orthodoxy in the mid-nineteenth century after a period of intense competition between rival practitioners (Inglis 1980). To be sure, there have been some recent signs of improvement in this fraught relationship, not least at a local, interpersonal level following the decision of the General Medical Council to drop its ethical prohibition on cooperation between doctors and alternative practitioners in the 1970s (Fulder and Monro 1982). However, the past tensions remain today at an institutional level, as epitomized by the scathing Report of the British Medical Association (1986) on alternative therapy which was largely negatively disposed towards unorthodox practices as they were not felt to match the standards of modern scientific medicine.

Interestingly, acupuncture was one of the more positively regarded types of alternative medicine in this Report, subject to the caveat that it be linked to medical practice for application to a limited range of conditions. This suggests that the reaction of the medical profession to each of the diverse range of therapies that make up alternative medicine may depend to some degree on the specific circumstances of the therapy concerned, which may alter over time. In this vein, Wardwell (1976) has argued that the medical response to particular alternative therapies will vary according to such factors as the extent to which they challenge the core assumptions of orthodox medicine; the numbers of their clientele; their political influence; the solidarity of the practitioner group; and the aspirations of the group in relation to the orthodox health care division of labour. As has been seen from the case of acupuncture, much of this framework may be applicable to the study of the response of the medical profession to alternative medicine in general in the British context.

This schema again, however, drives the inquirer back to a model of medical decision-making about alternative therapy based more on professional self-interests in the politics of health care than considerations of public responsibility. Whether this is reflected in the response of the medical profession to areas of alternative medicine other than acupuncture needs more thorough investigation, particularly given that not all alternative therapies can be considered equally safe and efficacious (Saks 1994). While questions can also be posed about the altruism of the medical profession in its reception of developments within the orthodox frame of reference itself (see, for example, Gould 1985; Collier 1989), it would be disconcerting in this context if the profession is not found to have adopted, or to be in the process of adopting, an approach to alternative medicine which is more in tune with its own self-proclaimed altruistic ideology – especially in light of the opportunities that are now beginning to open up for non-medically qualified alternative therapists to practise on a contracted basis within the new market-oriented National Health Service (Saks 1992a).

This point is sharpened by the sensitive situation that lies ahead for alternative therapies in Britain in the Single Market. With harmonization, the Single Market could have a major restrictive impact on the availability of alternative medicine in this country, where the freedom to practise such therapies is currently more extensive than in most other parts of Europe (Huggon and Trench 1992). Given that orthodox medical associations in Britain and elsewhere are likely to have a crucial influence on state decision-making within the European Community in this fast-changing field (Gaier 1991), it is particularly vital that such deliberations are entered into by the medical profession in this country with due regard for the implications for the wider public and not just for the parochial self-interests of those within the profession.

The question of the public interest orientation of the medical profession by implication also raises crucial issues about the potential role of the state in this area in the future – issues which are interestingly highlighted by the most recent Report of the British Medical Association (1993) on non-conventional therapies. Following the analysis of the situation of such therapies in Britain and the rest of Europe, this Report focuses more on seeking to ensure that adequate forms of state regulation of alternative therapies are in place in this country than on their condemnation *per se*. Appropriate modes of state regulation are indeed vital if the public interest is to be advanced in this field. However, the case of the medical response to acupuncture in modern Britain suggests that any public interest-inspired review of the state regulation of health care in this country may need to consider critically the advantages and disadvantages of the present state support for the dominant position of the medical profession within the health service, as well as the regulation of its largely disenfranchised unorthodox competitors.

REFERENCES

British Medical Association (1986) *Report of the Board of Science and Education on Alternative Therapy*, London: BMA.
—— (1993) *Complementary Medicine: New Approaches to Good Practice*, Oxford: Oxford University Press.
Bynum, W. F. and Porter, R. (eds) (1987) *Medical Fringe and Medical Orthodoxy*, London: Croom Helm.
Collier, J. (1989) *The Health Conspiracy*, London: Century Hutchinson.
Crompton, R. (1990) 'Professions in the current context', *Work, Employment and Society* May: 147–66.
Dearlove, J. and Saunders, P. (1984) *Introduction to British Politics*, Cambridge: Polity Press.
Department of Health (1989) *Working for Patients*, London: HMSO.
—— (1991) *The Patient's Charter*, London: HMSO.
Esland, G. (1980) 'Diagnosis and therapy', in G. Esland and G. Salaman (eds), *The Politics of Work and Occupations*, Milton Keynes: Open University Press.
Fulder, S. (1988) *The Handbook of Complementary Medicine*, Oxford: Oxford University Press.
Fulder, S. and Monro, R. (1982) *The Status of Complementary Medicine in the United Kingdom*, London: Threshold Foundation.
Gaier, H. (1991) 'Reveille for biocentric medicine', in G. Lewith and D. Aldridge (eds), *Complementary Medicine and the European Community*, Saffron Walden: C. W. Daniel.
Gould, D. (1985) *The Medical Mafia*, London: Sphere.
Huggon, T. and Trench, A. (1992) 'Brussels post-1992: protector or persecutor?', in M. Saks (ed.), *Alternative Medicine in Britain*, Oxford: Clarendon Press.
Inglis, B. (1980) *Natural Medicine*, Glasgow: Fontana.
Larkin, G. V. (1983) *Occupational Monopoly and Modern Medicine*, London: Tavistock.
Lewith, G. (1985) 'Acupuncture and transcutaneous nerve stimulation', in G. Lewith (ed.), *Alternative Therapies: A Guide to Complementary Medicine for the Health Professional*, London: Heinemann.
Lu Gwei-Djen and Needham, J. (1980) *Celestial Lancets: A History and Rationale of Acupuncture and Moxa*, Cambridge: Cambridge University Press.
Macdonald, A. (1982) *Acupuncture: From Ancient Art to Modern Medicine*, London: Allen & Unwin.
Mann, F. (1973) *Acupuncture: Cure of Many Diseases*, London: Pan Books.
Marshall, T. (1963) 'The recent history of professionalism in relation to social structure and social policy', in T. Marshall, *Sociology at the Crossroads and Other Essays*, London: Heinemann.
Moran, M. and Wood, B. (1993) *States, Regulation and the Medical Profession*, Buckingham: Open University Press.
Navarro, V. (1986) *Crisis, Health and Medicine: A Social Critique*, London: Tavistock.
Nicholls, P. A. (1988) *Homoeopathy and the Medical Profession*, London: Croom Helm.
Nicholls, P. A. and Luton, J. E. (1986) *Doctors and Complementary Medicine: A Survey of General Practitioners in the Potteries*, Occasional Paper No. 2, Department of Sociology, North Staffordshire Polytechnic.
Reilly, D. T. (1983) 'Young doctors' views on alternative medicine', *British Medical Journal* 287: 337–39.
Richman, J. (1987) *Medicine and Health*, London: Longman.
Robson, J. (1973) 'The NHS Company Inc.? The social consequences of the professional dominance in the National Health Service', *International Journal of Health Services* 3(3): 413–26.
Saks, M. (1985) 'Professions and the public interest: the response of the medical profession

to acupuncture in nineteenth and twentieth century Britain', PhD thesis, Department of Sociology, London School of Economics, University of London.

—— (1990) 'Sociology, professions and the public interest: professional ideology and public responsibility', paper presented at International Sociological Association Conference on Professions and Public Authority, Northeastern University, Boston, USA, 21–2 April.

—— (1991a) 'Power, politics and alternative medicine', *Talking Politics* 3(2): 68–72.

—— (1991b) 'The flight from science? The reporting of acupuncture in mainstream British medical journals 1800–1990', *Complementary Medical Research* 5(3): 178–82.

—— (1992a) 'Introduction', in M. Saks (ed.), *Alternative Medicine in Britain*, Oxford: Clarendon Press.

—— (1992b) 'The paradox of incorporation: acupuncture and the medical profession in modern Britain', in M. Saks (ed.), *Alternative Medicine in Britain*, Oxford: Clarendon Press.

—— (1994) 'The alternatives to medicine', in J. Gabe, D. Kelleher and G. Williams (eds), *Challenging Medicine*, London: Routledge.

Shao, Y. (1988) *Health Care in China*, London: Office of Health Economics.

Sharma, U. (1992) *Complementary Medicine Today: Patients and Practitioners*, London: Routledge.

Standen, C. S. (1993) 'The implications of the Osteopaths Act', *Complementary Therapies in Medicine* 1: 208–10.

Wardwell, W. (1976) 'Orthodox and unorthodox practitioners', in R. Wallis and P. Morley (eds), *Marginal Medicine*, London: Peter Owen.

Webster, A. J. (1979) 'Scientific controversy and socio-cognitive metonymy: the case of acupuncture', in R. Wallis (ed.), *On the Margins of Science: The Social Construction of Rejected Knowledge*, Sociological Review Monograph No. 27, Keele: University of Keele.

Wharton, R. and Lewith, G. (1986) 'Complementary medicine and the general practitioner', *British Medical Journal* 292: 1498–500.

8 The British General Medical Council
From Empire to Europe

Meg Stacey

This chapter examines changes in the regulation of doctors in Britain consequent upon the transition from empire to Europe, developing already-published work on the British General Medical Council (Stacey 1992). The history illustrates some points about the imbeddedness of professionals and their organizations in the society of which they are a part. Professions not only reflect that society's complexities, but are also in a sense determined by its history and by their own historical development within it. More than mirroring it, however, they continually contribute to the society's creation and change.

Amid the disputes as to what constitutes a profession, there is some agreement that professions are occupations whose members have undergone lengthy and systematic training; which are accorded some rights of self-regulation; control the standards of skill needed for entry to their occupation; and maintain members' discipline. In return they are accorded a privileged status among occupations. The notion of service to fellow members of the society is closely linked with the idea of profession; service freely rendered in return for an acceptable fee or salary. While so much may be agreed, there is a good deal more dispute as to whether such occupations fulfil their part of the bargain by providing trustworthy service or whether they misuse, in their own interests, the privileges they have been accorded.

Theorists of the professions have sometimes talked of the concept of profession as if professions are somehow the same wherever they are found or at least that there are certain characteristics which can be extracted regardless of time and place. There may be some truth in this. However, what is also important to note is the extent to which what a 'profession' is and what 'professionals' do is dependent on the social, economic and political circumstances in which that occupation finds itself.

In my understanding professions are occupations which have historically made a successful bid for this privileged status. In the case of medicine in Britain the close historical relationship between the rise of the profession and the rise of the bourgeoisie in the eighteenth and nineteenth centuries along with the development of industrial capitalism has been well documented (Jewson 1974; Inkster 1977; Larson 1977; Pelling 1978; Peterson 1978; Webster 1981; Waddington 1984; Porter 1987). There can be little doubt that the professions occupy particular positions in the class structure, and ones which are not static over time. The analysis by Larson (1977) of the rise of medicine in Europe and the United States demonstrates how many present professional practices were developed in past struggles to gain preference over other healers; she shows, too, how far the circumstances of modern medical practice, health care organization and economic arrangements have become removed from those early days when medicine defined itself as a profession. What has been less acknowledged or documented until recently is the gendered nature of the way in which professions developed (Clark 1968; Oakley 1976; L'Esperance 1977; Gamarnikow 1978; Versluysen 1980; Stacey 1981, 1988: chs 6, 8, 14–16; Davies 1983; Donnison 1988; Witz 1992). Even less sociological acknowledgement has been accorded to the way in which oppressive racial and ethnic relations have been built into some professional developments (but see Moss 1992).

The establishment of the European Community has demonstrated the manifold national differences among all the professions in the member states. As Orzack says: 'Differences in political traditions, educational history, applications of technology to practice, government styles, practitioner status, and association authority are profound' (1983: 252). The major sociological dispute as to whether the professions are a beneficent influence in society or are largely self-serving has in the past paid insufficient attention to these empirical differences. Freidson (1970a, 1970b, 1986) and Larson (1977) in the United States and Johnson (1972, 1977, 1982) in the United Kingdom are among those who focus on the control which professionals have over others in the division of health labour and over the client. Inheritors of the first, Durkheimian, position are Carr-Saunders and Wilson (1933) and more recently Dahrendorf (1984, 1991).

Dahrendorf, in origin a German, many years resident in the United Kingdom and one time European Commissioner, by no means ignores national differences in what professions are and can do. As a continental with early life experience of an oppressive totalitarian state he finds particular merit in what he calls the 'English professions' (Dahrendorf 1984) whose contract is with society rather than the state (but see Rueschemeyer 1989). He is greatly disturbed by the damage done, during the right radical regime in power in Britain throughout the 1980s, to the professions, and to other institutions intermediate between the state and the individual, institutions such as the universities (Dahrendorf 1991). I share Dahrendorf's anxiety at the weakening of these intermediate bodies, which also include the trade unions and local government. During those years we experienced the extraordinary phenomenon of the encouragement of the free market in the name of liberty but at the same time a frightening increase in the powers of the central state and commensurate reductions in individual and group liberty. In this situation one must be grateful for – and support – any strong organized group which may continue to stand between the individual and the state and when necessary oppose it, as medicine sometimes does.

When Dahrendorf speaks of liberty in this context he does not ask the question 'whose liberty?' His location of professions in the social arrangements of different countries is partial. He is concerned about the amount of autonomy professions have and how independent they are of the state. He is correct to draw attention to the important differences in Europe as to who actually regulates medicine, how close in some the state is to the registration and entry processes and how important it is to contemporary Eastern Europeans to have organizations independent of the state. The question 'whose liberty?', however, requires going beyond the political also to locate the professions in historically dynamic social, cultural and economic terms. This extension includes asking how well the professions fulfil their side of the bargain with society to provide a good service.

My detailed experience is with medicine. For nine years I was a lay member of the General Medical Council which regulates medicine in Britain, and I have subsequently studied it systematically. Historical evidence shows that the nascent medical profession in the nineteenth century persuaded the state to register certain qualified medical practitioners of which it approved (that is, the allopaths) and not others. The profession had entered into a contract with society to ensure that registered medical practitioners could be trusted to do a competent job (Merrison 1975). True to the libertarian British tradition, and unlike practice in many European countries, other healers were not thereby banned from practice; they simply could not call themselves 'registered medical practitioners'. Furthermore all state medical posts were reserved for registered practitioners, an increasingly important privilege as the state became more involved with health care.

My research sought to establish how, in exercising its regulatory function, the Council kept the balance between maintaining the unity of the profession (essential if an occupation is to regulate itself satisfactorily) and protecting the public. The evidence turned out to be that the profession came first, but a crucial research conundrum which emerged was the following: how could a group of such essentially decent and well-meaning men (mostly men) with high ethical standards fail to see they were not making a good job of protecting the public? The answer had to do with their historical and contemporary position in British society, deeply divided by status, class and 'race'.

Like all other associations, organizations and statutory bodies, the General Medical Council comes out of and is locked into the structure and culture of British society (see Vogel 1986; Brazier *et al.* 1994). It is composed of an élite body of people who are still predominantly male, white and status-striving middle class. The Council is part, albeit a minor part, of the ruling élites (or, if you prefer, ruling classes) of British society, élites which historically were associated with the rulers of the British Empire; élites which have now, since the break up of empire, thrown their hand in with Europe. These were the people who had to adjust to the free movement of labour in Europe, but who also had been used to drawing labour from the Empire.

In what follows I outline the reactions and behaviour of this group, the regulators of British medicine, in this transition from empire to Europe as it is encapsulated in the differential treatment of overseas-qualified and European-qualified doctors. First, however, I explain the General Medical Council briefly for those who are not familiar with it.

THE GENERAL MEDICAL COUNCIL: ITS CONSTITUTION AND FUNCTIONS

The General Medical Council is a statutory body set up originally in 1858 and currently governed by the Medical Act of 1983. It is, nevertheless, independent of the state and financed by the profession whose registration fees and annual retention fees constitute a main source of income. Other sources are fees charged for certain services. However, practitioners are entitled to claim the registration fee as practice expenses or against income tax. Until 1994, the Chief Medical Officer of England (a civil servant) sat as a Council member while the Chief Medical Officers of Scotland, Wales and Northern Ireland sat as members in rotation. However, after 1979, none of the Chief Medical Officers was permitted to serve on any committees: the profession's leaders guard its independence of the state jealously. As from 1 April 1994, the two Chief Medical Officers (for England and Wales) resigned their seats to make space for more lay members (see below, this page). The Chief Medical Officers may continue to attend *ex officio* as observers.

The essence of the powers of the General Medical Council, which are granted to it by Parliament, lies in its control of the registers of practitioners which it keeps and publishes. The Council controls entry to the registers by deciding what qualifications are necessary for registration. This it does by approving medical schools whose training and education are sufficiently in line with the guidance it offers as to the content of basic medical education. The guidance is established after thorough consultation with the medical schools and is not proscriptive; experimentation is encouraged. The General Medical Council may remove persons from the register temporarily or permanently if they have become unfit to practise. Such practitioners are discovered by examining reports of complaints or convictions made against them. The Council may visit and inspect medical schools, but since it has no inspectorate, it relies entirely on the reports received as to continuing competence to practise.

Members of the General Medical Council are drawn from three main sources: appointment by universities and Royal Colleges; election by registered medical practitioners of each of the four countries of the United Kingdom; and nomination by the Queen in Privy Council, which rather mystifying term really means in this context by the Health Ministers. Table 8.1 shows the constitution of the Council in 1992. It now has over 100 members and, since 1979, elected members have a constitutional majority over all others together. This is a prime route whereby rank-and-file doctors, particularly general practitioners, can gain a voice, but also whereby the British Medical Association, the doctor's major trade union, can influence Council policy and practice. The Privy Council nominees are a way whereby the state may exercise some influence. Until 1926, when the first layman [*sic*] was appointed, all these state nominees were medical. The General Medical Council now wishes the proportion of the lay to rise to a fifth by reducing the appointed members.

Women are still under-represented. In 1976, when I was first appointed, there

Table 8.1 Constitution of the GMC in 1992

Members	
Appointed by	
universities	21
Royal Colleges[1]	14
Total appointed	35
Elected by registered medical practitioners in	
England[2]	42
Scotland	7
Wales	3
Northern Ireland	2
Total elected	54
Nominated by Privy Council	
medical	2
lay	11[3]
Total nominated	13
Total members	102

1   Royal Colleges includes Faculties.
2   England includes the Channel Islands and the Isle of Man.
3   Includes one nurse and one pharmacist.

Source: General Medical Council (personal communication).

were only three women (two lay; one elected doctor) out of the then 46 total members. Since the Council was reformed and enlarged in 1979, there have been rather more, 11 by 1990, but still less than their proportion on the register. In 1976 no doctors came from ethnic minorities. Six were elected in 1979 from the nominees of the Overseas Doctors Association.[1]

As this brief summary shows, the General Medical Council differs from some regulatory bodies in continental Europe in two principal ways. First, the control of registration and of educational qualifications are united in one body along with the maintenance of discipline. Second, this body is independent of the state, although necessarily subject to state influence.

The centralized educational control at first only covered basic medical education. In 1950 control was extended to cover the 'pre-registration year', a year of supervised practice between qualification and graduation from medical school and being fully admitted to the register. Since 1979 the General Medical Council has had responsibility for coordinating all stages of medical education. It does not, however, have the same control over post-graduate education as it has over basic medical education. Post-graduate education is the responsibility of the various Royal Colleges and Faculties which determine when a doctor has satisfied them that she or he is qualified to be a specialist. Other post-graduate training bodies are also involved. The United Kingdom definition of what is a specialist differs from that in many countries of Europe and the training required is longer.

THE REGISTERS

To understand the issues around overseas and European doctors, the modes of registration of doctors in the United Kingdom have to be appreciated. On the *main register* (or principal list) are recorded those doctors granted *full registration*. British-educated doctors who have satisfactorily completed their medical school qualifying examinations are admitted to the *provisional register* while they undertake their pre-registration year. Satisfactory completion of this admits them to full registration.

The General Medical Council does not publish a specialist register, although the topic has been discussed since the mid-1970s. To comply with the European Community directive, a list of registered medical practitioners holding certain specialist qualifications is kept. Since 1990 after wide consultation qualified specialists may, but need not, indicate in the register any higher specialist training they have completed. Each Royal College maintains its own records of those who have gained and completed its qualifications.

Some arrangements have existed since 1886 for the registration of overseas-qualified doctors. In 1947 a category of *temporary registration* was introduced for doctors who wished to enter the country to practise for a short period – to gain post-graduate experience, for example. Presumably in recognition of a felt need for the continuing presence of overseas-qualified doctors to staff the National Health Service, the 1969 Medical Act took the 'temporariness' out of temporary registration, that is, those who applied no longer had to say they intended to leave the country in a defined period.

The General Medical Council recognized some overseas qualifications for full and provisional registration as providing a standard (and, although not spelled out in the Acts, a type) of medical education deemed appropriate in the United Kingdom. The qualifications recognized were mostly those given by medical schools founded abroad by United Kingdom doctors in the colonial empire where instruction was, initially at least, in English. Recognition was associated with reciprocity, so that United Kingdom-registered doctors were entitled to practise in countries where reciprocal arrangements applied – this arrangement was clearly of benefit in facilitating the mobility of medical practitioners within the Empire and later the Commonwealth. Government, through the Privy Council, was involved in establishing reciprocity with particular countries, but took General Medical Council advice. The Council arranged for the visitation of recognized medical schools, much of it informal; senior United Kingdom doctors who visited for another purpose would report on standards and conditions. In 1973, 86 schools overseas were recognized.

Doctors who qualify in *recognized* medical schools are accepted for *full registration* so long as they have verified clinical experience not less extensive than they would have gained in the United Kingdom pre-registration year. Those who lack this can apply for *provisional registration* and are only able to work in hospital house officer posts under supervision. Overseas doctors, not qualified for full registration because they held qualifications from unrecognized schools, could before 1979 apply for *temporary registration*. Qualifications in some 90 countries were in 1970 recognized for temporary registration. Doctors so registered were licensed to practise only in specific appointments in hospitals approved by the General Medical Council. Registration for one such post after another was the mode. In 1974, 6,897 doctors were temporarily registered under these arrangements, but in that year 13,777 periods of temporary registration had been granted. Such doctors could become fully registered by obtaining the diploma of the Royal College of Surgeons and the Royal College of Physicians, the licentiate of the Society of Apothecaries of London, or the joint qualification of the Scottish Royal Colleges. Overseas doctors, like those qualified in the United Kingdom, paid registration fees. In 1973 this was a one-off £10 for provisional and £35 for full registration for the latter with a £2 retention fee. Temporary registration cost overseas doctors £5 for two months or less, £10 for two to 12 months and £5 per 12 months thereafter.

TRADITIONS OF PREJUDICE

Restriction of entry is, of course, of the essence in occupations claiming to be professions. Sometimes restriction is exercised not only against those lacking appropriate qualifications, but also using other considerations – although these may be dressed up in terms of inappropriateness. The British register was used for many years to keep women out of medicine, even when they were qualified, by denying their qualifications (medical schools also refused to admit them) (Scott 1984, 1988). National boundaries are another such example which the Treaty of Rome was designed to overcome so far as Europe was concerned. Professionals, in common with members of any occupation, tend to be more restrictive where national rivalries are involved, especially when large numbers of incomers seem to threaten jobs (see Orzack 1983: 252; 1991: Conclusions). Racism as well as nationalism may be involved.

Organized British medicine, regrettably, does not have a reputation for openness or generosity in the admission of foreign doctors to its numbers, although Professor Dahrendorf suspects that its record 'is at least as good as, say, the French, let alone the German' (personal communication 1993). The history of the treatment meted out to refugees, Jewish and non-Jewish alike, from Nazi Germany and from Austria has yet to be fully written. The story (remembered with pain by those who went through it) is now beginning to be put together and published (Berghahn 1984: 83–7; Weindling 1991; Dr David Pyke currently has a study in hand). The emerging story redounds to the discredit of British medicine.

While medical scientists were supportive and worked to find places for Nazi refugees in their laboratories, medical practitioners were restrictive. The United Kingdom thereby lost much good service which could have been immediately available in under-doctored parts of the country. British practitioners also lost the opportunity to learn from the medical knowledge and practice the refugees brought with them, some of it much more advanced than was available in Britain at the time. Some medical practitioners who were refused registration moved on to other countries where they were able to re-establish themselves as practising professionals; others were never again able fully to use their skills. Qualified and experienced German and Austrian practitioners had to struggle to retrain to satisfy the General Medical Council so that they might practise. When medical person-power became short in the Second World War some were admitted to a specially established temporary war-time Register, but this only permitted very restricted practice.

THE NHS AND OVERSEAS DOCTORS

After it was established in 1948, the National Health Service, with its service free at the point of delivery, revealed a demand for health care that could not be met by the number of doctors that British medical schools could supply. In theory a number of solutions to the problem were possible, for example training nurses to take greater responsibility or training a further category of doctor's assistant. But suspicious as British practitioners were of doctors trained elsewhere, the medical view seemed to be that qualified practitioners were always preferable to the lay (in British usage 'lay' includes all non-medical health care practitioners). However that may be, doctors from abroad and particularly from the Indian sub-continent were encouraged to come and work in British hospitals. They came in considerable numbers.

In 1974 the government health departments reported 8,000 young doctors qualified overseas in training grades in the NHS, 42 per cent of the total (Merrison 1975). Most would return home later. Allowing for this, maintenance of the development of the National Health Service (still then expanding) required the annual admission of between 2,500 and 3,000 doctors from overseas. United Kingdom medical schools in 1973 produced 2,289 doctors. In 1974 the number of overseas doctors practising in the United Kingdom was still increasing, although expected to decline as the output of the United Kingdom medical schools, including the new schools, increased (Merrison 1975: 58–9). The register tells a similar story: in 1938 about one-twentieth of registered medical practitioners had qualified in ex-colonial or foreign medical schools; by 1972 the proportion had risen to one-third (General Medical Council's evidence to Merrison).

This dependence on so many overseas doctors had caused trouble; trouble among the public and trouble within the profession. While it was not the main cause of the Merrison Inquiry being set up – that was due to a professional revolt (see Stacey 1992) – the registration of these doctors had come to be seen as a major problem. The temporary registration arrangements were cumbersome and inappropriate for such large numbers, tedious for the doctors, their employers and the General Medical Council. The British public, even those not overtly racially prejudiced, were unused to being treated by non-white doctors; the linguistic skills of many were claimed to be insufficient, making doctor–patient communication inadequate for proper diagnosis and treatment. Some medical and nursing staffs made similar complaints and also questioned clinical competence. The Merrison Committee reached what it called 'the inescapable conclusion . . . that there are substantial numbers of overseas doctors whose skill and care . . . [falls] below that generally acceptable in this country, and it is at least possible that there are some who should not be registered'. The division of responsibility between government and General Medical Council was to blame; the Council had allowed 'its duty as the protector of medical standards to be compromised by the manpower [*sic*] requirements of the NHS' (Merrison 1975: paras 185, 187).

Faced with lay and professional complaints about the large influx of overseas doctors in the 1960s, the General Medical Council – even before the Merrison Committee was appointed – had in 1971 set up its own inquiry. This consulted widely but included no overseas-qualified practitioners, nor were there any on the Merrison Committee. The close links of senior United Kingdom doctors with the recognized hospitals had loosened since ex-colonial territories achieved independence; some schools were now teaching in indigenous languages; privately General Medical Council members distrusted the integrity of some of the examination processes.

ACTION TO CONTROL STANDARDS

Although the Council's 1971 Committee had – in the absence of documented evidence to the contrary – concluded that very few overseas doctors whose professional knowledge had been seriously deficient had been granted registration, it nevertheless advised greater control (GMC *Minutes* 1972). One solution was to reduce drastically the number of the foreign medical schools the General Medical Council recognized. The process continued throughout the 1970s. Of 90 schools recognized in 1970 only 23 were left in 1976, reduced to 21 by 1982 but rising to 22 in 1984. From 1981 universities wishing to maintain their recognition had to make annual returns.

Changes in the registration procedures followed the Merrison Inquiry. The Council had rejected the idea of a test such as that imposed by the United States Education Council for Foreign Medical Graduates and Merrison agreed. The subsequent 1979 Medical Act, following the advice the Council itself made to the Merrison Committee, instead replaced *temporary* by *limited registration*. Registration ceased to be attached only to one post. Council had discretion as to the period for which registration would be granted, although there would be no residence time limit, and discretion also as to the range of employment that could be undertaken. Universities whose qualifications were not recognized for full registration could apply for the recognition of their courses for limited registration.

Merrison recommended that all doctors practising in Britain should have a qualification which the General Medical Council could recognize as comparable to that of a doctor trained in the United Kingdom. The Council anticipated the legislation. It quickly sought and gained confirmation from government that it would not be illegal to test the linguistic and clinical competence of applicants for temporary registration. It set up a new body in 1974 to manage these tests, the Temporary Registration Assessment Board, independent of but linked with the Council. When temporary became limited registration, the Temporary Registration Assessment Board was changed to the Professional and Linguistic Assessment Board.

Initially the assessment was based on a comprehension test of spoken English; a multiple choice question paper to test factual professional knowledge, covering medicine, surgery and obstetrics; a test of written professional English – 'a modified essay question'; and a *viva voce* examination to test practical professional knowledge as well as proficiency in English. The tests continually evolved throughout the first decade of their use. For example, simulations of clinical situations were added and later other additions made to substitute for a full clinical examination – this remained impracticable on logistic and financial grounds (*GMC Annual Report for 1987*). In 1988 a more modern English comprehension test was added. Candidates have to pass all the components of the examination at the same sitting. Many took the test again and again, never managing to pass all components at once. So many doctors were taking the test four times or more that Council decided that from 1981, if a doctor failed a test severely after three attempts, she or he would be refused further attempts.

Other routes to limited registration exist for those without recognized qualifications. A sponsorship scheme admits overseas doctors, by prior arrangement, to a training post under the tutelage of a consultant or similar senior doctor in the United Kingdom willing to provide and supervise their training. This scheme has been used increasingly since 1980 and by 1987 was reported as becoming of greater importance than the Professional and Linguistic Assessment Board test.

Doctors from abroad who lack qualifications entitling them to full registration may, having practised under limited registration for a specified period and being able to produce evidence of an appropriate record, be accorded full registration: a committee is designated for this purpose. Alternatively, they may re-qualify in the United Kingdom. Finally, full registration is temporarily granted to a small number of visiting specialists.

MORE BRITISH DOCTORS

The influx of doctors from abroad in the 1960s and 1970s was associated with National Health Service staff shortages: the aim then was to control but not staunch the flow. By 1980 the tide was turning: graduates from the new United Kingdom universities were in the market. Fear of medical unemployment again arose, although some areas and some specialties were still short-handed, such as geriatrics and psychiatry, for example, where overseas doctors had been disproportionately employed (Smith 1980; Anwar and Ali 1987). Nevertheless, by 1980 the profession as a whole began to view the continued influx of overseas doctors in an even more reserved manner than hitherto.

Committee minutes, particularly the comments made to overseas doctors facing discipline, suggest that the Council's attempts to control immigrant doctors became increasingly tough at the beginning of the 1980s. When the Council's Overseas Committee felt it had the situation under control utterances became more beneficent; this was after the 1985 change in immigration rules to restrict doctors to a four-year permit-free stay in the United Kingdom. The effect of this would prevent the full use of the five years limited registration which the 1978 Medical Act allowed – causing anxiety and upset to overseas doctors who might be required to go home before achieving full registration.

Over a period of fifteen years or so thousands of young doctors had come from countries with different life-styles, different arrays of common presenting complaints, and different economic and social security systems. Given this it would have seemed reasonable to have made induction and orientation courses available to the incomers, but this was not done. The actions taken were all restrictive: no attempt was made to help the incoming doctors over these problems which were not precisely medical and could not necessarily be said to come under the normal practice of supervising consultant or senior registrar. There is no evidence to suggest that the General Medical Council made any recommendations for such positive actions, nor did the Department of Health or National Health Service authorities make any provision. Yet how much the National Health Service owed to these doctors was frequently reiterated by the authorities.

While all this was going on and increasing restrictions were being put into place, the drama in relation to European Community-qualified doctors had already begun. In medical regulation old imperial links were ending and Europeanism beginning. Since, as indicated above, the Nazi oppression and the ethics of free science had not been enough to open the doors of the medical profession to the refugees, it is perhaps understandable that the free mobility of labour promised in the Treaty of Rome was something of an alien idea. When it became clearer that this mobility would be orchestrated by directives ('directive' has a menacing quality to libertarian Anglo-Saxon ears) from elsewhere over which British professional bodies would have little control, the prospect was seen by many as positively alarming.

THE FIRST MEDICAL DIRECTIVES

The new regulations relating to immigrant doctors were proposed by the General Medical Council in 1973; the Merrison recommendations were published in 1975; the Medical Act was passed in 1978. The United Kingdom had joined the European Community in 1972, but this was not confirmed until the referendum of 1975. Nevertheless in 1972 the General Medical Council's Executive and Education Committees began discussing the possible effects for medical regulation in Britain of the draft medical directives designed to ensure the free mobility of labour throughout the European Community. The two directives (75/362/EEC; 75/363/EEC) were adopted by the Council of Ministers in June 1975 to become effective by December of 1976, although the United Kingdom government was unable to make the necessary legislative changes until June 1977, producing an awkward interregnum for the Council. Thus, shakily, a new era began for the regulation of medicine in the United Kingdom and, for the General Medical Council, a new and reduced status.

A number of factors caused the Council anxiety. First of all it could not itself deal directly with the European Community authorities as it did with British Ministers and civil servants. It had to work through the British government which had decided, given the multiplicity of bodies with authority over British medical practitioners (for example, the Royal Colleges, Faculties and various joint committees), that only it could express an overall United Kingdom view in European Community deliberations. As time went by, government was able to nominate General Medical Council representatives to certain European Community bodies.

A second concern was that the delayed entry to the European Community had meant that the United Kingdom had not been fully engaged in the preliminary discussions about the draft medical directives, largely agreed before the United Kingdom joined (for a brief account of the early days of the medical directives, see Orzack 1980). The General Medical Council felt, as the Registrar put it, the directives 'substantially reflect the organization and structure of medical practice in the continental states' (*GMC Annual Report for 1976*: 9).

Then there was the timing – just when controls on overseas doctors were being increased. The potential contradiction in tightening controls on doctors coming from the Commonwealth – in practice, particularly those from the new Commonwealth – at the same time as controls on doctors from European Community countries were to be removed or loosened was obvious. This had two aspects: first, the loss of General Medical Council control over who practised medicine in the United Kingdom; and, second, the political embarrassment.

LOSS OF CONTROL: LANGUAGE AND CLINICAL SKILLS

The Registrar made the point clearly when he said:

It is interesting to compare the concept of free movement in the EEC with the traditional arrangements for 'reciprocity' with other countries. Since 1886 there has been a substantial traffic both outwards and inwards under these arrangements. This system of reciprocity has always involved a positive act of recognition by Council of overseas qualifications. By contrast the obligations of this country under the EEC Treaty are based primarily on political decisions. The Council has virtually no discretion as to which qualifications granted in member states it must accept and register.

(GMC Annual Report for 1976: 11)

The Merrison Committee (Merrison 1975) had welcomed the mutual recognition of medical qualifications within the European Community but hoped that means would be found to ensure that the same fitness to practise rules would apply to European Community- as to United Kingdom-qualified doctors and that 'incoming doctors are both familiar with English and with professional ethics and practice in the UK'. These standards Merrison recommended should apply to overseas doctors and should, where necessary, be ensured through linguistic and clinical tests.

Two factors led to the political embarrassment: first, the unequal treatment of European and overseas doctors; second, the right under European Community rules for British doctors to move freely in Europe while non-British, but British-registered, doctors could not. Doctors from ex-colonial territories, who already felt exploited within the National Health Service, saw this as yet another discrimination against them.

COPING WITH THE CHANGES

The General Medical Council reacted in two ways: first, by seeking to retain as much control and authority over medical practice in the United Kingdom as possible; second, by trying to influence medical developments in the European Community. In terms of retaining control, given the ongoing problems with the influx of overseas doctors, a first aim was to try to ensure that the European doctors it registered had appropriate linguistic and clinical skills. The General Medical Council also wished to be designated as the 'competent authority' for necessary administrative tasks, such as registering European Community practitioners and issuing certificates of equivalence and certificates of completion of specialist training. In terms of influencing medical developments and control of standards in Europe, the Council encouraged the establishment within the European Community of the Advisory Committee on Medical Training. It became worried when it thought it might not have a seat on that body – which it in the end was granted. Council has placed much importance on its work on that committee (see Brearley 1984).

THE LANGUAGE QUESTION: SOLUTION AND CHALLENGE

The Council persuaded the British government that it should be given some control over the standards of incoming European Community doctors – government was vulnerable to the same embarrassment as the General Medical Council about the standards of the incomers. The consultative document issued in 1976 by the Department of Health and Social Security on the implementation of the medical directives proposed powers for the Council 'to examine in appropriate cases the linguistic knowledge of doctors from other member states who come to practise here and if necessary to defer registration until they are satisfied that an appropriate degree of linguistic knowledge has been achieved' (quoted in GMC *Minutes* 1976 CXIII App. IX: 266). The document further suggested that the Temporary Registration Assessment Board (later Professional and Linguistic Assessment Board) tests should be used for this purpose. The Council had already gained the agreement of the Temporary Registration Assessment Board to accept this responsibility and to devise appropriate tests for European incomers.

The Medical Qualifications (EEC Recognition) Order, finally made in 1977, provided, among other things, that any national of a member state applying for full registration in the United Kingdom had 'to satisfy the Registrar, on or after registration that he [*sic*] has the necessary knowledge of English'. It gave the Council powers to provide tests of English (GMC *Minutes* 1977 CXIV App. III: 171), but not for clinical tests. Testing started at once. In the first nine months of 1977 26 European Community doctors took a language test, of whom 20 passed, including two who had passed at the second attempt; six failed.

Hardly was this arrangement in place than it was challenged. Other member states complained at the meeting of the Committee of Senior Officials in Public Health in November 1977. The Commission was involved and two visitors were sent to the United Kingdom in November and December 1978. The General Medical Council was told in 1979 that the Commission was considering legal action against the United Kingdom. (See Orzack 1980: 11–7——11–8 on the clear precedence given in Europe to European Community citizens' right to practise anywhere in the European Community over against their linguistic skills.) Government, judging that the chances of the United Kingdom winning any case brought were small, suggested a compromise the Commission would support which involved abolishing the statutory requirement of linguistic proficiency as a condition of registration.

> Instead NHS bodies would require EEC doctors who wished to work in the NHS to produce evidence of the knowledge of English required for the particular work they would be doing. Tests of English language ability could be made by a number of means. An Order in Council would be prepared to make the necessary changes in the existing law and advice would be given to NHS authorities by circular.
>
> (GMC *Minutes* 1980 CXVII: 68)

On 1 August 1981 testing ceased. From then until 1983 the Council continually asked the Department of Health and Social Security to ensure that National Health Service employing authorities checked the proficiency of incoming European Community doctors. Thereafter all mention in the GMC *Minutes* and *Annual Reports* of the linguistic proficiency of these practitioners ceased.

This controversy took place against a background in which the English translation of the relevant directive included the words that the governments of member states 'shall see to it' that doctors from other European Community countries have an adequate knowledge of the language of the country where they want to practise. The United Kingdom had not been entirely alone in its anxiety about the competence of incoming European Community doctors: the Germans had raised the matter in 1970 and are said to have returned to the issue (Rowe, personal communication 1992).

A LANGUAGE PROBLEM TODAY?

The General Medical Council confirmed that in its understanding in the United Kingdom incoming European Community doctors are required to satisfy the authorities by whom they are employed as medical practitioners in the UK, that their proficiency in written and spoken English is sufficient for that employment. If the employing authorities are not satisfied of a doctor's linguistic competence, they can advise the doctor to take a test . . . in essence, if the linguistic skills of a doctor are questionable the employing authority should not engage the doctor for that employment.

(GMC, personal communication 1992)

Wondering how matters were handled in the National Health Service, I wrote in February 1992 to the managers of each of the fourteen English Regions (apologies to the other three countries). After explaining my purpose, I said: 'I write now to ask what arrangements there are in your Region for ensuring that registered medical practitioners from Europe have sufficient linguistic skills to treat the patients they are expected to attend. And also whether you feel the arrangements are satisfactory?'

Of the fourteen Regions, thirteen ultimately replied, of which five took the trouble to consult with their District Health Authorities. At the time of inquiry, generally speaking, registrars, consultants and associated specialists were employed by the Region, a teaching hospital or newly formed National Health Service trusts. Others, mostly more junior, were taken on at district level or by trusts. The replies, which came sometimes from the managers and sometimes from a personnel or manpower [*sic*] planning officer on the manager's behalf, are very varied. They show a good deal of doubt and confusion and differing levels of thoughtfulness.

Ten Regions said specifically and another implied that they applied no linguistic tests. Three mentioned no check they make (or advise districts to make); the remaining ten relied mainly on interviews: three mentioned interviews alone; two interviews and pre-interviews or pre-interview visits. One mentioned an informal rotational scheme with specific European hospitals where reliance is placed upon a recommendation and visit. Another which does some recruiting in Europe uses clear job specifications.

Most authorities appeared to feel that interviews and pre-interviews revealed linguistic skills sufficiently well; however, four mentioned cases where linguistic weakness had emerged later. None mentioned this as being so bad that appointments had to be terminated, although one reported language problems preventing a doctor moving on to a senior house officer post. Three Regions said, as one put it, 'one or two doctors have given some concern in the first month or so of their appointments'. Another specifically regretted that the authority did not apply a test of idiomatic English, an area where weakness might not be revealed in interview, but important when communicating with patients. The purpose of such a test would be to offer the doctor further training if necessary.

Three Regions overtly recognized their responsibility to ensure that a doctor's linguistic skills are appropriate for the post for which she or he is applying. In some others I had the sense that this was not the case. Two clearly felt that to suggest tests to applicants would be illegal; in one case because further qualifications cannot be required of incoming European Community doctors and would be tantamount to 'racial discrimination'; the other feared contravening equal opportunities legislation. In contrast, two other authorities were clear that where language is important for a post and is so specified it would be legal to test it before appointment. Three indicated that they specified appropriate linguistic skills as necessary in the job description, thus ensuring they were on firm ground in exploring linguistic as well as clinical skills.

One authority simply felt there was considerable difficulty in this area, had unresolved problems and asked for any guidance that might be available. Indeed a number of regions specifically asked to have access to any helpful information I might come across. One indicated that while they did not have problems now, if there were any large influx of doctors from Europe then problems might arise.

The General Medical Council told me that 'since 1981, very few EC doctors have actually applied to take the test, and in recent years the number has decreased considerably . . . in 1991 there were . . . no more than six' (GMC, personal communication 1992). No records are kept as to whether these doctors took the test voluntarily or were advised to do so by a potential employer. The fee for the Professional and Linguistic Assessment Board English test in 1992 was £220 with a £150 cancellation fee: perhaps the low number of doctors taking the test is not surprising. In the past two years the General Medical Council had received reports from two employing authorities where language problems have been encountered.

The Department of Health issued guidance about European Community doctors and their knowledge of English in June 1987. Authorities were notified in June 1990 that that guidance will continue to apply until June 1996 when it will be reviewed. This guidance was inspired by concern on the part of the General Medical Council and the Department of Health about a 'small but significant number of overseas qualified doctors eligible for limited registration who continue to work in [NHS] hospitals outside the terms of the conditions specified on their Certificate of Limited Registration or without any form of registration at all' (Department of Health PM(87)7: 1) and is mostly concerned with that problem. It does, however, include four paragraphs about doctors qualified in the European Community who 'are entitled to full registration with the GMC'. The guidance continues:

> The Department recommends that when considering the appointment of an applicant to an NHS post, including that of a locum, the employing authority should satisfy itself that the doctor's knowledge and use of English is such as to enable him [*sic*] properly to perform the duties of his post. In order to assess this, authorities may interview the applicant personally or require evidence of linguistic competence, making it clearly understood that such information is necessary to satisfy the authority that the needs of the particular post will be adequately met.

The Department of Health also indicates that reference may be made to competence in English so long as the information 'is clearly relevant to the needs of the particular post'. Issues to do with erasure or suspension from the register (with regard to which European Community doctors are treated like United Kingdom doctors) are also referred to.

Given the doubts expressed in the Regions and the Districts about the legality of linguistic tests, I asked the Department of Health for further clarification and received the following response:

> There is no reason why employing authorities should not offer their own tests so as to satisfy themselves that an applicant for a job would be able to fulfil the needs of the posts applied for. The linguistic component of the PLAB test or other tests could *only* be required where there is no other way of ensuring that the applicant has the necessary linguistic ability. Where, for example, an interview or academic qualifications held by the applicant indicated satisfactory knowledge of English then it would not be appropriate to ask the applicant to undergo [a formal test].
>
> (Department of Health, personal communication 1992; original emphasis)

In the light of this, the varied interpretations of and caution about the legal situation expressed by the Regions are not perhaps surprising. One further comment: other informants have pointed out that in districts where there are sizeable minorities of specific European nationals, the presence of a European Community doctor who speaks that language can be very valuable.

WHAT THE PATIENTS SAY

Given the unease some Regions reported and the apparent vagueness of control mechanisms, I asked patient-oriented organizations whether they had had any reports of language difficulties. The Association of Community Health Councils of England and Wales said it had no complaints from its constituent bodies, although it was aware that some health authorities did not even check properly whether doctors they were employing were registered with the General Medical Council. Inquiries of Community Health Councils at the district level would be needed to be sure patients have no problems, but the Association would have heard of anything major. Neither had the Patients Association received any complaints about European doctors of which linguistic skills were a part. Apparently there is no problem, it has not surfaced or it is handled informally locally. Furthermore, problems, if there are any, may not emerge where only a few patients are involved.

THE IMPORTANCE OF NUMBERS

Analysing the General Medical Council and Europe in 1984, Roger Brearley concluded: 'medical migration, the main expected effect of community membership, has proved to be unimportant' (1984: 1363). The fears of an influx had not been fulfilled and little difficulty was felt. Senior doctors confirm this is still true. Collectively the situation is not threatening and a few juniors can be helped individually. The small numbers are in great contrast to those of overseas doctors who have been employed in the United Kingdom.

Table 8.2 shows the slow start: up to 1988 in no year did the number qualified in European Community countries other than Britain who were granted full registration rise to 1,000. This compares with the peak year for overseas doctors, 1976, when nearly 7,000 were on the temporary register. The cumulative total in 1992 for European Community registrations was 8,823, a known overestimate since some will have withdrawn their names: the number remaining is not reported.

QUALITY OF PRACTITIONER

Numbers are discussed in the General Medical Council when new countries join the European Community. Some member states do not control the numbers of

Table 8.2 European Community and overseas intakes compared

Year	EC fully registered		Overseas qualified	
	No. added each year	*Total* [1]	*Full*	*Limited* [2]
1974	0	0	1,930	6,897
1975	0	0	2,741	–
1976	0	0	3,133	6,912
1977	85	85	2,800	6,555
1978	109	194	2,669	5,982
1979	124	318	1,814	4,339
1980	134	452	3,771	5,544
1981	184	636	1,497	5,308
1982	264	900	1,165	5,077
1983	327	1,227	1,369	5,928
1984	302	1,529	1,696	5,582
1985	332	1,861	1,869	5,085
1986	445	2,306	1,707	4,586
1987	995	3,301	1,915	3,876
1988	1,309	4,610	1,753	4,986
1989	1,184	5,794	2,183	5,546
1990	1,020	6,814	2,118	6,434
1991	956	7,770	2,689	6,577
1992	1,053	8,823	2,365	7,877

1 A cumulative total from which some will have removed their names (numbers unknown).
2 Temporary registration until 14 February 1979 when limited registration begins. Some apparent discrepancies appear in the reported numbers. Wherever possible those cited in the text of the relevant year have been used.

Source: GMC *Minutes, Annual Reports* and personal communication 1993.

practitioners produced; the General Medical Council is dubious about medical education in others. In 1981 Spain, Portugal and Greece caused anxiety; the founder member, Italy, has been a constant source of worry. Relief is expressed that member states are now trying to limit their medical school intakes. The United Kingdom with much more restricted numbers of doctors per head of population is afraid of becoming 'a haven' for unemployed doctors from countries about whose standard of medical education the General Medical Council is suspicious.

Some countries are seen to be 'more different from us' than others, for example the Mediterranean countries, whose nationals are also sometimes said to be more likely to have language problems. British doctors working on European bodies are increasingly coming to recognize that different does not necessarily mean worse or wrong.

Some European doctors working in the United Kingdom feel our practices discriminate against them. This led to the formation in December 1992, of the European Doctors Association at a meeting held in the Spanish Chamber of Commerce in London. The prime mover was a Spanish specialist and, according to the *Lancet* (1992), Spaniards and Italians formed the bulk of the founding audience. There are echoes here of the founding of the Overseas Doctors Association, with the very important difference that the European Doctors Association is Europe-oriented and has representatives in a number of European countries.

WHAT IS AND WHO ARE SPECIALISTS?

The collision in 1992 over specialist qualifications, when the European Community again threatened legal action, relates to the General Medical Council's limited powers over post-graduate medical education, in turn derived from the continuing power of the Royal Colleges, the oldest of which antedate the General Medical Council by 300 years. The present problem goes back fifteen years, but the immediate precipitating factor was the General Medical Council's 1990 decision mentioned earlier to allow practitioners who had completed their United Kingdom specialist qualifications to indicate this in the register by adding 'T'. Completed specialist training varies among the colleges but implies longer and more advanced training than the European Community-required designation 'specialist'. The European Community considers the 'T' listing may discriminate against specialists from other European countries (Brearley 1992: 662). The European Community challenge also has to do with the United Kingdom's system of issuing certificates of specialist education. While the General Medical Council is the competent authority in European Community terms to do this, it has relied upon the Royal Colleges and the associated joint training committees (whose criteria are not consistent one with another) for advice on each candidate (Brearley 1992: 661).

The relationship between post-graduate and basic medical education has caused the General Medical Council difficulty for many years. It has lacked statutory power to control the situation (see Stacey 1992: 115–23; 241–3). The

Department of Health responded to the European threat by setting up a working party to advise Ministers on these problems, including the standards required in the United Kingdom for consultant appointments, opening up a hornet's nest of discontent about consultant posts and the entire structure of the division of medical labour, itself deriving from the pattern originally established through the Royal Colleges. The recent Calman Report has taken a grip of the problem which effectively overrides the General Medical Council and the colleges – implying changes in British medical regulation.

CONCLUSION

This chapter has addressed medical aspects of the United Kingdom transition from an imperial power to a European nation. This involves moving from a dominating relationship of power, authority and control to one of equal partnership. The granting of dominion status to erstwhile colonies implied a largely equal partnership, but it was not granted to all ex-colonies and not all of them accepted that option. Relationships with other member states in the European Community are necessarily of equal partnership and fully reciprocal; citizens of those states are to be treated as similarly free and equal persons as are British citizens.

A necessary change has been from direct control to one of influence only. British medical leaders, no less than other British élites hitherto in positions of authority at home and to some extent overseas, experienced the transition as painful. This transition from control to influence emerges in the comparison of the treatment of 'overseas' and European incoming doctors. Initially the General Medical Council, backed by the British government, attempted to exert a similar control over Economic Community doctors as they had over other foreigners. In this they failed.

The General Medical Council's aim to become the competent authority for the administration of the United Kingdom side of control of professional qualifications has only partly succeeded. The directive on specific training in general medical practice which was approved in 1986, for implementation in 1995, owed much to the efforts of British general practitioners, who, in the absence of such a directive, had their recently achieved United Kingdom status as a specialty at risk in the European arena. Not everything which the British wanted was achieved, but the directive is seen as an advance. However the British government has insisted that the General Medical Council share the competent authority status with regard to this directive with another body, the Joint Committee of Postgraduate Training. Furthermore, as we have seen, the Council's execution of its task as a competent authority with regard to specialist certification has been challenged and government has had to intervene. The Council's status is subject to change from pressures at home as well as from the European Community. Transition to Europe has unleashed and strengthened these.

ACKNOWLEDGEMENTS

Initial work on the General Medical Council was grant-aided by the ESRC (GOO232247); a Leverhulme Emeritus Fellowship helped the preparation of this chapter, providing research assistance given by Dr Phil Moss. My gratitude is expressed to him, to both funders and to the many private individuals and officials who helped with information, understanding, interpretation and criticism. Special thanks are also due to Mrs Margaret Truswell for her secretarial services and Jennifer Lorch for her help. However, only I am responsible for any errors of fact or judgement and for the opinions which are expressed here.

NOTE

1   The use of the term 'overseas' is peculiar. While technically it describes anyone from outside our island shores, in practice it is often given a narrower meaning and is used particularly in relation to the old colonial territories. In the case of 'overseas-qualified doctors' the term has effectively come to be applied to those doctors from the 'New Commonwealth' and Pakistan, but also from other countries, whose medical status is thought to be similar, for instance some in the Middle East. The 'Old Commonwealth' is made up of countries such as Canada, Australia and New Zealand which have predominantly Caucasian populations. Recognition of their training schools rarely raised problems, although there are no reciprocal relations with Canada, at Canada's request. The 'New Commonwealth', on the other hand, comprises those countries with a predominantly black- or brown-skinned population. 'Overseas' is consequently a pejorative, indeed racist, term. I use it because it is the term in official use in the General Medical Council and applied particularly to doctors from abroad whose skills are tested before they may be registered, not all but many of whom come from the ex-colonial territories. The term was reclaimed by some of the overseas doctors themselves in the formation of the Overseas Doctors Association, predominantly of Asian-qualified doctors, to protect and improve their status in the United Kingdom by joint action.

REFERENCES

Anwar, M. and Ali, A. (1987) *Overseas Doctors: Experience and Expectations*, London: Commission for Racial Equality.

Berghahn, M. (1984) *German-Jewish Refugees in England: The Ambiguities of Assimilation*, London: Macmillan.

Brazier, M., Lovecy, J. and Moran, M. (1994) *Professional Regulation and the Single European Market: A Study of the Regulation of Doctors and Lawyers in England and France*, University of Manchester, mimeo.

Brearley, R. (1984) 'Medicine in the European communities', *British Medical Journal* 17 November: 1360–3.

Brearley, S. (1992) 'Specialist medical training and the European community', *British Medical Journal* 19 September: 661–2.

Carr-Saunders, A. M. and Wilson, P. A. (1933) *The Professions*, Oxford: Clarendon Press.

Clark, A. (1968) *Working Life of Women in the Seventeenth Century* (1st edition, 1919), London: Frank Cass.

Dahrendorf, R. (1984) 'In defence of the English professions', *Journal of the Royal Society of Medicine* 77: 178–85.

—— (1991) In the broadcast discussion *Analysis* on the threat from the general manager to the professions, presented by David Walker, produced by Simon Coates, BBC Radio 4, 7 November.

Davies, C. (1983) 'Historical explanations of the contemporary division of labour in child health care', in M. Stacey and C. Davies, *Division of Labour in Child Health Care: Final Report to the SSRC*, Coventry: University of Warwick.

Donnison, J. (1988) *Midwives and Medical Men: A History of Inter-professional Rivalry and Women's Rights*, 2nd edition, New Barnet: Historical Publications.

Freidson, E. (1970a) *Profession of Medicine: A Study in the Sociology of Applied Knowledge*, New York: Dodd Mead & Co.

—— (1970b) *Professional Dominance: The Social Structure of Medical Care*, New York: Atherton.

—— (1986) *Professional Powers: A Study of the Institutionalization of Formal Knowledge*, Chicago: University of Chicago Press.

Gamarnikow, E. (1978) 'Sexual divisions of labour: the case of nursing', in A. Kuhn and A. M. Wolpe (eds), *Feminism and Materialism*, London: Routledge & Kegan Paul.

Inkster, I. (1977) 'Marginal men: aspects of the social role of the medical community in Sheffield 1790–1850', in J. Woodward and D. Richards (eds), *Health Care and Popular Medicine in Nineteenth-Century England*, London: Croom Helm.

Jewson, N. (1974) 'Medical knowledge and the patronage system in eighteenth-century England', *Sociology* 8: 369–85.

Johnson, T. J. (1972) *Professions and Power*, London: Macmillan.

—— (1977) 'The professions in the class structure', in R. Scase, (ed.), *Industrial Society: Class, Cleavage and Control*, London: Allen & Unwin.

—— (1982) 'The state and the professions: peculiarities of the British', in A. Giddens and G. Mackenzie (eds), *Social Class and the Division of Labour: Essays in Honour of Ilya Neustadt*, Cambridge: Cambridge University Press.

Lancet (1992) 'European Doctors Association', *Lancet* 12 December: 1463–4.

Larson, M. S. (1977) *The Rise of Professionalism: A Sociological Analysis*, Berkeley: University of California Press.

L'Esperance, J. (1977) 'Doctors and women in nineteenth-century society: sexuality and role', in J. Woodward and D. Richards (eds), *Health Care and Popular Medicine in Nineteenth-Century England*, London: Croom Helm.

Merrison, A. W. (1975) *Report of the Committee of Inquiry into the Regulation of the Medical Profession*, London: HMSO.

Moss, P. (1992) 'The migration and racialization of doctors from the Indian sub-continent', unpublished PhD thesis, University of Warwick.

Oakley, A. (1976) 'Wisewoman and medicine man: changes in the management of childbirth', in J. Mitchell and A. Oakley (eds), *The Rights and Wrongs of Women*, Harmondsworth: Penguin.

Orzack, L. H. (1980) 'Educators, practitioners and politicians in the European Common Market', *Higher Education* 9: 307–23.

—— (1983) 'International authority and national regulation: architects, engineers, and the European Economic Community', *Law and Human Behaviour* 7(213): 251–64.

—— (1991) 'The General Systems Directive: education and the liberal professions', in L. Hurwitz and C. Lequesne (eds), *The State of the European Community: Politics, Institutions and Debates in the Transition Years 1989–90*, London: Longman.

Pelling, M. (1978) *Cholera Fever and English Medicine 1825–1865*, Oxford: Oxford University Press.

Peterson, M. J. (1978) *The Medical Profession in Mid-Victorian London*, Berkeley: University of California Press.

Porter, R. (1987) *Disease, Medicine and Society in England 1550–1860*, London: Macmillan.

Rueschemeyer, D. (1989) 'Comparing legal professions: a state-centred approach', in R. Abel and P. Lewis (eds), *Lawyers in Society: Comparative Theories*, Berkeley: University of California Press.

Scott, J. (1984) 'Women and the GMC', *British Medical Journal* 22 December: 1764–7.
—— (1988) 'Women and the GMC: the struggle for representation', *Journal of the Royal Society of Medicine* 81: 164–6.
Smith, D. J. (1980) *Overseas Doctors in the National Health Service*, London: Policy Studies Institute.
Stacey, M. (1981) 'The division of labour revisited or overcoming the two Adams', in P. Abrams and R. Deem (eds), *Practice and Progress: British Sociology 1950–1980*, London: Allen & Unwin.
—— (1988) *The Sociology of Health and Healing: A Textbook*, London: Unwin Hyman.
—— (1992) *Regulating British Medicine: The General Medical Council*, London: John Wiley.
Versluysen, M. (1980) 'Old wive's tales? Women healers in English history', in C. Davies (ed.), *Rewriting Nursing History*, London: Croom Helm.
Vogel, D. (1986) *National Styles of Regulation*, Ithaca, New York: Cornell University Press.
Waddington, I. (1984) *The Medical Profession in the Industrial Revolution*, Dublin: Gill & Macmillan.
Webster, C. (ed.) (1981) *Biology, Medicine and Society: 1840–1940*, Cambridge: Cambridge University Press.
Weindling, P. (1991) 'The contribution of central European Jews to medical science and practice in Britain, the 1930s–1950s', in E. M.Werner (ed.), *Second Chance: Two Centuries of German-speaking Jews in the United Kingdom*, Tübingen: J. C. B. Mohr (Paul Siebeck).
Witz, A. (1992) *Professions and Patriarchy*, London: Routledge.

References to General Medical Council *Annual Reports* and *Minutes* (published by the General Medical Council, London) are cited in the text.

Part III

Health professions and the state in continental Europe

9 The politics of the Spanish medical profession
Democratization and the construction of the national health system

Josep Rodríguez

The organization of health care in Spain is undergoing major transformations. Most of these stem from changes that have taken place throughout the last two decades (Linz *et al.* 1982). The end of the Franco period and the consolidation of a democratic system frame the political transformation of the health system (Maravall 1982). The creation of the *Sistema Nacional de Salud* (National Health System) integrates the processes of change within the system and shapes the current health care complex. The medical profession has also undergone an important change in its structure and political role during these years. For decades, the profession has been a dominant force in defining and controlling the nature of medical work (de Miguel 1976). The transformation of medical care into health care inevitably leads to changes in the political role of the profession, having to share its influence and power with government regulators and corporate and insurance interests. This modification is guided by the revaluation of both state intervention in health care and the political dominance of the profession in designing the organization of the system. The process of transition in the health care system is taking place within a major transformation of Spanish society and its political system (Ministerio de Sanidad y Consumo 1984). New social values and priorities concur with the construction of a new political system and new mechanisms of political intervention.

PROFESSIONAL WORK IN THE 1980S

A distinctive element of the practice of the Spanish medical profession is the complexity of its work, with professionals combining several practices and institutional settings. This complexity is the result of the process of adjustment between the development of the medical profession and that of the health care system (Nadal 1984). Using survey data (Centro de Investigaciones Sociológicas 1983) an accurate map of the adjustment and accommodation among the various types of practice (for example, private, public, in complex hospital organization and in less complex settings) can be built which configures medical work. It also explains the mechanisms through which the profession is to some extent able to escape bureaucratizing and proletarianizing tendencies (implicit in the great development of the Spanish public health care system) and is able to maintain a large liberal and private practice.

In spite of the great dependency of the medical profession on public administration, almost 40 per cent of its professional practice still takes place in the private sector (see Table 9.1). And in spite of the large development and dominance of the hospital system, almost 66 per cent of medical work still takes place outside the hospital. The private practice of medicine occurs largely outside the hospital system, while public practice is split between the hospital and much less complex organizations and settings. It is worth noting that over 18 per cent of medical work is completely liberal (autonomous) and totally independent from any institutions (either public or private). Public medical work is mostly organized while private work is mainly in solo form (either liberal or related to health insurance). In terms of organizational complexity, the work of the Spanish medical profession is split into three main types of practice: a third in very complex organizations (public and non-profit hospitals), a third in simple and slightly bureaucratized organizations (public primary health centres and out-patient facilities), and a third in private offices. This situation slows down the strong pressures to transform the profession into a bureaucratized employee occupation. While this tendency is dominant in the hospital structure, its strength is limited in the primary health and ambulatory centres. These are smaller and much simpler organizations, without strong hierarchical structures, which in some respects resemble associative forms of practice. In overall terms, the profession's level of autonomy, especially at the clinical level, is still very high: it has counterbalanced the strong tendency to employment status (82 per cent of its work) and its dependency on the state (62 per cent of its practice) by keeping a considerable part of its work within limited levels of bureaucratization and external control.

This articulation of the main and secondary professional practices provides us with a good indicator of the system of relations which generates the complexity of medical work. Public practice has been shrinking (in relative terms) since 1973 as a result of the slowdown in the development of the public sector (see Table 9.2). This reduction is compensated by an increase in hospital public practice. This corroborates the previously shown trend (de Miguel and Guillén 1987; Rodríguez 1987) towards the construction of a public health care system

Table 9.1 Distribution of medical work (%)

	Public sector	Private	Liberal practice	Total
Hospital	30.7	4.1	–	34.8
Out-patient services	29.4	1.5	–	30.9
Individual practice	3.6	11.9	18.7	34.2
Total	63.7	17.5	18.7	100.0

Source: Centro de Investigaciones Sociológicas (1983).

Table 9.2 Changes in the main practice of medicine, 1979 and 1983 (%)

	1979 [1]			1983 [2]		
	Public	*Private*	*Total*	*Public*	*Private*	*Total*
Hospital	25.1	3.7	28.8	38.8	4.4	43.2
Extra-hospital	54.3	16.8	71.1	34.3	22.5	56.8
Total	79.4	20.5	100.0	73.1	26.9	100.0

Source: 1. Servicio de Estudios Sociológicos del Instituto de Estudios de la Seguridad Social (1979); 2. Centro de Investigaciones Sociológicas (1983).

based increasingly on the hospital system. In spite of such trends, medicine is still mainly practised within the public system (almost 75 per cent) and more than half (56 per cent) is practised in non-hospital settings. Fifteen per cent of the main professional practice is totally liberal and independent office-based, and an additional 11 per cent is in solo practice associated with or dependent on private institutions. In total, one-quarter of mainstream medical practice is still individual in form. The state, through either its central structure (*Instituto Nacional de la Salud*[1]) or its local and regional health structures (since 1987 integrated into the National Health System [*Sistema Nacional de Salud*] along with the *Instituto Nacional de la Salud*), is the principal agent in the construction of organized medicine. While the practice of medicine in the private market is clearly individual, in the public sector it is organized (see Table 9.3).

Forty-eight per cent of the profession has at least one second practice. The parameters of this second practice are radically different from the main practice. They complement each other in a singular and peculiar process of accommo-

Table 9.3 Distribution of main professional practice by institutional setting and ownership (%)

	Hospital	*Ambulatory*	*Private office*	*Total*
Social security	25.3	24.8	1.7	51.8
Central administration	8.3	4.0	1.5	13.8
Local and regional administration	5.6	1.4	0.3	7.3
Non-profit organizations	1.4	–	0.2	1.6
For-profit organizations	2.7	0.7	7.6	11.0
Private office	–	–	14.5	14.5
Total	43.3	30.9	25.8	100.0

N = 1,032

Source: Centro de Investigaciones Sociológicas (1983).

dation. The chief practice is mainly within the organized public sector. The secondary practice takes place in the private sector (52 per cent) and also individual settings (49 per cent). Totally autonomous practice accounts for almost one-quarter of the total of this secondary practice. Although the main practice takes the form of bureaucratized employment, the complementary practice seems to ensure the special status of the profession: it provides it with the possibility of practising medicine in an independent manner, as it has been socialized as a liberal profession.

The Spanish medical profession, or at least a large portion of it, has been able perfectly to combine in its development over the past five decades increasing employment in large public organizations depending directly on the state with a high level of work in the private market and especially in solo/individual practice. This combination is the result of collaboration with the state during the years of construction of the public system (*Instituto Nacional de la Salud*) and it differentiates the profession from that of other countries. This work/practice arrangement is the direct result of the status of medicine as a public profession, that is to say, it both works for the public sector (mainly the state) and is endowed by the state with the responsibility and power to design and control its professional work and organization (the health care system).

The Spanish medical profession is a collective split into two groups: those that combine public with private practice and those limited to the status of public employees. One is a group that, even though it also has employee status, maintains the characteristics of a liberal profession. The other group is being progressively proletarianized. The profession itself is articulated as a class system. Type of practice and specialization are the dominant classificatory elements. Being mainly an employee in the public system and in generalist specialties shapes the most proletarian part of the profession. Having positions in the system associated with important individual practices and the most prestigious specialties are the characteristics of the upper class of the profession. Physicians coming from the lower classes will more likely move into the 'lower-class' profession while those coming from the upper classes will move into the 'upper class' of the profession.

The structural characteristics of the profession are basic to understanding the configuration of its professional interests and its orientation towards the practice of medicine. The structural elements to single out are: its dependent development with respect to the creation of the health care market around the public system; professional practice dependent on the state; geographical concentration in the richest areas and in large cities; split practice between hospital and non-hospital settings; its status as a public profession; the combination of practice as employee in complex organizations with liberal practice; and the split in the profession between those who combine public and private practice and those employed and closer to proletarian status. The ongoing corporatization of medicine in Spain (to a large extent the result of the liberalization measures adopted in the 1990s by the socialist administration) is leading the profession towards proletarianization and at the same time is reducing its share in the private market and its opportunities for individual liberal practice.

The history of the profession has shaped its political personality, and even its own conception as profession. The medical profession was forced to participate in the *Seguro Obligatorio de Enfermedad*[2] and politically co-opted through compulsory affiliation into the Official Medical Association (whose leaders were appointed by the Ministry of Interior). This double dependency (political and professional) made it difficult for the profession to articulate any type of interests. The authoritarianism of the association system, until then prevalent, and the lack of discussion and exchange of ideas within it, are factors which have sped up the growth of ideological factions within the profession (Martín López 1979).

The development of organized medicine has produced substantial changes in professional parameters. The last fifty years have witnessed a complete transformation in the medical-health care market and in the role of the profession in it. It has moved from medicine practised in a liberal way to health care produced by complex organizations that use the services of different health professionals (physicians among them). Hospitals have become the central organizations in the provision of health care services, and directly employ and organize the work of almost half the profession (Rodríguez 1987). Of the 43 per cent of professionals working in primary health care, approximately half of them work in organized structures (although with high levels of 'autonomy'): outpatient services (*ambulatorios*) and primary care centres (*centros de salud*). The traditional practice of medicine, in which there is a direct contractual doctor–patient relationship, has been reduced to less than one-fifth of the total professional market (Guillén 1987).

Professional services are now the responsibility of health care organizations which are in charge of organizing the provision of medical services and of satisfying the demand for them. Originally that demand was exclusively for medical services, but with the expansion of health care organizations, and the transformation of what were once medical services into health care services, it has been channelled into a demand for a health care product. Although the profession still offers the same professional product, the market for it is no longer formed solely by the public but is determined by the health care organizations. The medical product is no longer sold for direct consumption but is integrated into a final health care package.

The supremacy of organized health care forces the profession to depend for its sustenance on organizational demand and to acquire employee status with no control over the demand for its own services. The dominant role of the state among the health care organizations transforms the employee status of the professional even more and practically turns him/her into a 'civil servant'. The supremacy of highly organized health care and the control of the state over the medical market is the main axis around which professional practice now turns (Pérez Díaz 1982).

Although the development of the Spanish medical profession has implied that an increasingly larger part of the profession centres its practice in hospital organizations, its participation in the complex structure of these organizations has diminished over time (Guillén 1987). Hospital organization evolves according to its own dynamics and little by little stops being the profession's exclusive domain. The organization develops its own needs and turns into an institution in which the medical profession, although it still has some power and autonomy, is clearly increasingly dependent on professional administrators.

PHYSICIANS AND SOCIAL CHANGE

A large part of the Spanish medical profession accepts public supremacy in the health care system because until recently this arrangement has made it possible for the profession to arrange its practice almost as it wanted (Instituto de Estudios de la Seguridad Social 1979; Centro de Investigaciones Sociológicas 1983). It was able to engage in private and liberal practice; and what is more important, it has been able to combine public with private practice. One of the main results of the transformation of the medical profession into a public profession has been its ability to maintain a great deal of its characteristics as a liberal profession. Nevertheless, advocates of radical changes are present in the profession. As a matter of fact, not only would some sectors of the profession like to change the overall organization of the system, but large sectors also support the enlargement of the private market, even under the supremacy and rule of the state, and total freedom in professional practice. In moments of political change, as the 1980s were in regard to health reform and as the beginning of the 1990s were in relation to counter-reform, it is important to understand what the forces of change within the profession are. It is precisely during these periods of transformation that opinions and positions become more polarized towards forms of organizational and professional practice close to the liberal model and the market, or towards socializing and proletarianizing models. In order to study the profession as a political actor we should understand the variables that explain its political positions with respect to health care reform.

To understand the forces dividing the medical profession in relation to the privatization or socialization of both the health care system and professional work, we have used SAS's logistic regression procedure. As dependent variables we have used dummy variables representing key structural features in professional practice and in professional careers. Entrance into the market before (or after) 1975 splits the profession into two clear groups: those who were able to take advantage of the development of the system, and as a result are well established and successful; and those entering the profession in moments of crisis and having to face either marginal positions in the market or unemployment. Being mostly a masculine profession until very recently, gender is also a key factor in explaining different positions in the professional career. Two of the most important variables we have found in explaining differences among professionals (and to a large extent responsible for the main split of the profession) are having a primarily liberal practice (as opposed to being employed) and being able to combine several practices (as opposed to being limited to only one job).

Table 9.4 presents the results of SAS's logistic multiple regression procedure for several models: wanting to change the overall organization of the system;

Table 9.4 Logistic multiple regression: professionals and social change

	Change in health care model			No change		
	Beta	*Chi-square*	*p*	*Beta*	*Chi-square*	*p*
Before 75 (After 75)	.4626	10.04	.0015	–	–	–
Sex: Male (Female)	–	–	–	–.4314	.866	.0033
Liberal (Employed)	.3797	5.92	.0419	–	–	–
Combination (Only one)	–	–	–	–.3884	6.17	.0130

Model chi-square: 38.34 4DF P: .00000 R: .143

	Socialization of health care			Privatization of health care		
	Beta	*Chi-square*	*p*	*Beta*	*Chi-square*	*p*
Before 75 (After 75)	–	–	–	.6707	15.27	.0001
Sex: Male (Female)	–	–	–	.5048	4.08	.0433
Liberal (Employed)	–	–	–	.5744	12.20	.0005
Combination (Only one)	–.8479	9.52	.0020	.5494	11.79	.0006

Model chi-square: 24.06 4DF P: .0001 R: .153   Model chi-square: 94.45 4DF P: .00000 R: .260

Before 75: Entering in market before 1975 (or after); Combination: Combination of several practices (or only one).
Liberal: Independent practice in main employment (or salaried work).

Source: Centro de Investigaciones Sociológicas (1983).

favouring either privatization or socialization of the system; supporting or opposing an increasing role of the private sector in the provision of public services; and being in favour or against limitations in the number of professional practices. The positions of professionals in the professional market and career explain the ideological division of the profession. Having entered the professional market before 1975, being male, being primarily involved in liberal practice, and combining several jobs or practices characterize the group of the profession with a liberal and privatizing orientation. Entering the profession in times of crisis, being female, being an employee, and having only one job are the characteristics of the group associated with defending public supremacy in health care and a model of a profession close to employee status.

A liberal or employee professional status and entering the profession before or after 1975 explain in a statistically significant way the support or rejection of changes in the organization of health care. Liberal professionals and those with more years in practice are in favour of changes while younger and mono-employed professionals are opposed to them. The four independent variables are statistically significant and have positive effects in explaining support for privatization. The strongest influence on privatization is seniority in the profession followed by liberal practice and a combination of several jobs. On the other hand, support for the socialization of the system is explained by mono-employment alone. While the main variables defining a large sector of the profession enter into play in explaining support for privatization, the defence of socialization is exclusively determined by employed positions in the profession.

The three variables which characterize a large part of the professional structure (year of entrance in the profession; liberal or employed status; and several jobs or mono-employment) have significant effects in explaining the support or rejection of wider participation by the private sector in the provision of public services (that is to say, wider participation in the National Health System). The effects of the three variables are positive and very similar in respect of support for a larger role for the private sector. By contrast, in accounting for the defence of the exclusive role of the public system in the provision of public health care, the effect of having only one job is more important than the other two variables. Again, more marginal and proletarianized positions explain the radical left positions.

The more radical sectors of the profession (mostly mono-employed) advocate the organization of health care with full-time public employment, and with no possibilities of other forms of professional practice. These professionals defend a model of professional practice as employees. The more conservative sectors of the profession, especially those with more years in the profession, defend a totally liberal professional model. This model implies that they have the opportunity to organize their work according to their own criteria; that is to say, practise medicine as they want and as much as they want to. Given state supremacy in health care and the fact that most professionals are public employees, the possibility of having other jobs or practices outside public medicine is vital in order to maintain their status as liberal professionals.

Professional success, measured in our case by having some liberal practice and combining two or more jobs, is the variable with strongest impact in shaping a large part of the collective action of the profession. In the case of the Spanish medical profession success is related more to the possibilities of combining public employment with liberal or private practice than with income *per se*. The medical profession splits into two main groups according to differences in practice: those combining liberal practice with public employment and those who are only employed.

In Table 9.5 we present the impact of the main structural variables on agreement (or disagreement) with the political behaviour of the health organizations and political institutions. The group in the profession with liberal practice as their main activity and those combining several practices, largely as a result of their entrance in the market during periods of fast development of the health care system, strongly support the political activity of the conservative professional organizations: the Official Medical Association and the *Confederación Española de Sindicatos Médicos*. Professionals limited to only one employment and normally younger offer support, although not as strongly, to the political activity of the left organizations: *Federación de Asociaciones para la Defensa de la Sanidad Pública* and class-oriented labour unions (the *Comisiones Oberas* which is communist-oriented and the *Unión General de Trabajadores* which is socialist-oriented). Given the character of medicine as a profession which still has a strong liberal component, the identification with and support given to these radical organizations is much weaker than the support given to the conservative ones. Having only one employment (in a professional situation close to conventional employment) or combining several practices is the variable which most strongly explains how the profession identifies with the organizations representing its interests.

In Table 9.6 we present the logistic regression model which accounts for the impact of structural variables on affiliation to professional organizations. Affiliation to the main professional union (*Confederación Española de Sindicatos Médicos*) is mainly determined by belonging to the cohorts entering the profession (and the health market) before 1975 and to a lesser extent by combining two or more practices. To be affiliated to class-oriented labour unions (the *Comisiones Oberas* and the *Unión General de Trabajadores*) is mainly explained by having entered the profession after 1975. As was pointed out earlier, there are two opposed union approaches. The *Confederación Española de Sindicatos Médicos* defends the interests of those professionals accommodated in the system during periods of growth who wish to maintain acquired work privileges and professional status.

The professional segments with marginal and very proletarianized positions in the market are very close to the traditional class-oriented union approaches defended by the *Comisiones Oberas* and the *Unión General de Trabajadores*. Affiliation to the left professional organization *Federación de Asociaciones para la Defensa de la Sanidad Pública* is explained by gender and type of work arrangement. Being female and having only one job are significant explanations

Table 9.5 Multiple regression: agreement/disagreement with political agenda of medical organizations

	OMC	CESM	FADSP	CCOO	UGT
Before 75 (After 75)	-.16865**	-.17812**	.10207*	.11326*	–
Sex: Male (Female)	–	–	–	–	–
Liberal (Employed)	-.10762**	-.12241*	–	–	–
Combination (Only one)	-.32807***	-.25228***	.32287***	.18670**	.17411**
R^2	.2340	.1775	.1735	.0869	.0731

* = $p < .05$; ** = $p < 001$; *** $p < 0001$

Before 75: Entering in market before 1975 (or after); Combination: Combination of several practices (or only one).
Liberal: Independent practice in main employment (or salaried work).

Organizations: OMC: *Organización Médico Colegial* (Offical Medical Association).
CESM: *Confederación Española de Sindicatos Médicos* (Main professional union).
FADSP: *Federación de Asociaciones para la Defensa de la Sanidad Pública* (Radical medical association).
CCOO: *Comisiones Obreras* (Labour union, communist tendency).
UGT: *Unión General de Trabajadores* (Labour union, socialist tendency).

Source: Centro de Investigaciones Sociológicas (1983).

Table 9.6 Logistic multiple regression: explaining professional affiliation

	CESM			CCOO–UGT		
	Beta	Chi-square	p	Beta	Chi-square	p
Before 75 (After 75)	1.01037	10.17	.0014	-1.17185	11.42	.0007
Sex: Male (Female)	–	–	–	–	–	–
Liberal (Employed)	–	–	–	–	–	–
Combination (Only one)	.618924	4.29	.0384	–	–	–
Model chi-square: 28.84 4DF P: .0000 R: .244				Model chi-square: 16.76 4DF P: .0021 R: .184		

	FADSP		
	Beta	Chi-square	p
Before 75 (After 75)	–	–	–
Sex: Male (Female)	-1.330485	8.00	.0047
Liberal 1 (Employed)	–	–	–
Combination (Only one)	-1.027589	4.65	.0311
Model Chi-square: 29.35 4DF P: .0000 R: .330			

Before 75: Entering in market before 1975 (or after); Combination: Combination of several practices (or only one).
Liberal: Independent practice in main employment (or salaried work).

Organizations: CESM: *Confederación Española de Sindicatos Médicos*
FADSP: *Federación de Asociaciones para la Defensa de la Sanidad Pública*.
CCOO: *Comisiones Obreras*.
UGT: *Unión General de Trabajadores*.

Source: Centro de Investigaciones Sociológicas (1983).

of affiliation to the *Federación de Asociaciones para la Defensa de la Sanidad Pública*. Younger physicians in marginal labour positions are the ones who articulate their action through radical left organizations.

The political and union action of the profession is strongly influenced by those structural variables dividing the profession into two main groups for collective action: those advocating a conception of the profession in which liberal practice stands side by side with public employment; and those defending a conception of the profession as salaried workers. In spite of the importance of this second group, the first orientation still has more support in the profession and much more capacity to mobilize professionals. The commitment to conservative organizations is stronger than identification with those organizations defending a 'proletarianizing' project. The growing relevance of the 'proletarianizing' approach, as a result of the fast-developing salarization of the profession, sharpens not only the confrontation between the profession and the state in relation to professional status, but also the internal conflict over the supremacy of one approach and one type or other of organization representing the profession.

The first decade of the new democratic era has been marked by the high level of political confrontation between the profession and the state. In overall terms, the confrontation has been characterized by the strong pro-liberal (and pro-private) positions of the profession and the expansionist will of the state (Ministerio de Sanidad y Consumo 1984; Organización Médica Colegial 1985). The political scene over these years, dominated by attempts to shape the future Spanish health care system, has been marked by two important political debates. The first one revolves around the model of health care organization; that is to say, around the limits and structure of the medical health market and the forms of medical practice. This debate has centred on two legal instruments regulating professional practice: *Ley de Incompatibilidades* (Work Incompatibility Act) and *Ley General de Sanidad* (Health Care Act) (Mansilla 1986). In its confrontation with the administration of the state (with socializing positions) the medical profession has been able to maintain the existence of private and liberal practice (although under public tutelage). In the second debate the struggle between the two approaches (that of the state and that of the profession) has moved to the terrain of the structure of the health care organizations. At stake is the authority of the profession to organize its own work, and its strategic position and power in organizations as well as the whole system. This political confrontation reveals the lack of adequate channels for the articulation of the interests of intermediate sectors of society and evidences the difficulties of a traditional democratic system in the resolution of conflicts. In this concrete case the formal democratic system was unable to develop mechanisms to resolve the confrontation between the medical profession and the state (Rodríguez 1992).

Shaping the whole political debate and confrontation we find the problems of a (traditionally) liberal profession rapidly moving away from liberal characteristics. The medical profession is losing some of the most valued elements of any profession: the capacity and authority to organize its own professional work. To this we should add those problems related to the loss of professional autonomy and independence, resulting from its integration into the organized structure of the welfare state. The political life of the profession is marked by the social supremacy of political conceptions which stress the union dimension of politics and which, as a result, undervalue and de-legitimize the articulation and defence of professional interests. The Spanish medical profession is confronted with a double challenge: to maintain at a minimum level its characteristics and values as a liberal profession and to be able to articulate its professional and political interests in a political arena dominated by a conception of politics as the defence of the global interests of society which precludes and does not legitimize sectorial interests and their representation.

THE POLITICS OF THE MEDICAL PROFESSION

In 1949, as part of its fascist 'social revolution', the Franco regime started the construction of what later would become the National Health System (*Sistema Nacional de Salud*). From that moment on, the state took the initiative and monopolized the design and construction of the medical market and the health care system. The state forced the medical profession into the public market and started shaping a public profession. At the beginning of this process the medical profession was completely reluctant to lose its liberal status and become a public profession but the political coercion and the enormous benefits it started receiving (plenty of secure jobs and ample opportunities to organize the health care organization and its own practice) soon ended its initial resistance. The creation of the Official Medical Association, with compulsory affiliation, was initially designed as a mechanism for political control of the profession. It aimed at ensuring professional participation in the social security health care system, at suppressing the articulation of alternative ideologies within the profession, and at preventing conflict with the state. As a reward the *Organización Médico Colegial* was endowed with public corporative status; that is to say, with the political capacity and legitimacy to represent the entire profession in its consulting relations with the state. The system at that time fitted well with the definition by Schmitter and Lehmbruch (1979) of 'state corporatism'.

The state created a large health care system and a compulsory public insurance scheme that eventually covered and offered health services to 99 per cent of the Spanish population. The very large development of the public health care system has facilitated very high levels of development for the profession. The growth of the Spanish medical profession reached levels not attained by any other European medical profession; and definitely much higher than the levels it might have arrived at in a privately dominated health care system. Over the decades, the growing public sector offered secure jobs and income for all professionals. As an intrinsic part of the corporatists' public relationship with the state, the medical profession became a public profession. It worked almost completely for the state and received from it a large part of the control over the design of the new public health care system (Rodríguez 1990).

With such political control, the profession was able to design the characteristics of the system, the social organization of work, and the features of professional practice. In designing the system, the new health care was based on curative medicine (the set of skills monopolized by the profession) rather than preventive medicine. Following professional ideology, the new health care system promoted specialization and the creation of large and technically well-endowed hospital structures and almost totally disregarded areas not so prestigious and not related to the scientific development of medicine (non-hospital and family medicine). The great influence and power the profession exerted over the system marked its clear professional orientation. Health care was defined as an organization providing professional services. The idea of professional service was seen as incompatible with cost-oriented and productivity criteria.

The profession's influence over the social organization of work resulted in loose work relations and a status closer to consultant than employee. It was able to influence the characteristics of professional practice, succeeding in building a framework that combined secure jobs in the public system with a large liberal/ independent practice, which complemented the failure of the public system in primary medicine. Its special 'liberal-consultant' status not only allowed physicians to exert a great deal of control over their own practice but for decades it was also very functional for their individual practice interests. The loose working relations of many physicians have hindered the rational organization of work in the public system which in turn has reduced the capacity of the system to respond properly to the large and always expanding demand. As a result part of such demand has been guided towards their own private and individual practices (de Miguel 1979).

Both the political and economic transitions the country has undergone over the last fifteen years have had important effects upon the profession. As part of the political change the public corporative status of the Official Medical Association was questioned both by the government and by the profession itself. Soon after the democratic transition, the Official Medical Association started to attempt to create its own political role independent from the state. While the Official Medical Association was trying to articulate independent political represent-ation, other sectors of the profession, due to the Official Medical Association's failure to represent their interests properly, started to create their own vehicles of representation. Professional-union interests found a representational mechanism in the newly created *Confederación Española de Sindicatos Médicos*. Left-wing socializing professional interests became represented by the *Federación de Asociaciones para la Defensa de la Sanidad Pública* and radical labour union interests by traditional labour unions (the *Comisiones Oberas* and the *Unión General de Trabajadores*). This process has represented the end of the Official Medical Association's representational monopoly. On the conservative side the *Confederación Española de Sindicatos Médicos* has replaced the Official Medical Association in the representation of work-related interests. Coinciding with the division of interests there is also the struggle over representation between the conservative side of the profession (the Official Medical Association and the *Confederación Española de Sindicatos Médicos*) and the left-wing side (the *Federación de Asociaciones para la Defensa de la Sanidad Pública*, the *Comisiones Oberas* and the *Unión General de Trabajadores*). The conservative side has defended a more traditional conception of the profession (with a large liberal status) and advocated the extension of the private market. The left-wing side has a salaried-proletarianarized view of physicians and has strongly defended the further socialization of health care. This internal political conflict has aggravated the profession's conflict over representation with the state. Especially during the period of office of the socialist governments (from 1982 onwards) there has been a continuous struggle between professional interest organizations and the state to articulate a new political role for the profession. The socialist party in government has broken corporative relations with the profession and refused to build any other kind of political relations. A large part of the conflicts during the 1980s therefore had a common cause: the conflict over the political role and channels of political participation of the profession.

The breakdown of political ties between the socialist government and the profession was a part of the process of total reorganization of the health care system in which the medical profession had little by little been deprived of some of the work privileges acquired during the previous decades and had lost control over the organization and design of the system to be replaced by government regulators and managers (Saturno 1987). This situation was also the direct result of the weakening of its bargaining power due to the oversupply of physicians produced during these years by the educational system (over which the profession has never had any control). Professional rationality has lost jurisdictional ground to economic rationality. This change in the rationality of the system has threatened the profession's status and work arrangements built during the development of the public system. Government regulations imposing full-time employment, preventing the combination of practices within the public system, regulating the work of physicians, and rationalizing public organizations were some of the measures aimed at transforming professional status and practice. As result of the attempts to replace professional by rational-managerial criteria the medical profession also lost its jurisdictional domain in designing the organization, functioning and product of the health care system. Its professional service/product, over which it exerted a high level of control for decades, is starting to merge into a broader health care organization and service over which the profession does not have as much control.

The economic crisis suffered by the country since the mid-1970s and the later attempts to revitalize the economic system have shifted the priorities of the welfare state (Ortún and Segura 1983). Social policy and services are most affected by the change in priorities and have suffered the largest budget reductions. The high rate of unemployment and the increase in retirements have also affected the distribution of public financing. The social security budget did not increase proportionally to the growing needs it attempted to solve (unemployment benefits, growing pensions and the health care coverage of the entire population). Given the acuteness (unemployment) and novelty (retirement) of the new 'social problems' a fast-growing part of the social security budget has been spent on unemployment benefits and pensions. The health care budget has not grown proportionally, in spite of the large increase in the size of the population covered, and as a result the expansion of the public health care system has been halted. The stagnation of the public health care market, along with a not very dynamic private market, has created problems of employment for the large supply of physicians. The replacement of professional criteria by economic rationality in the organization of the system has resulted in the substitution of the objective of expansion by the objective of maximization of existing resources. As a result not many new jobs have been created, which in turn has further aggravated the problems of the employment of the profession.

The arrival of the Socialist Party (*Partido Socialista Obrero Español*) to power in 1982 radically changed the professional political dynamics. The official organization of the profession was deprived of substantial areas of its public corporative status which led to a systematic confrontation with the state. The main issues in the dispute between the profession and the government have been over the articulation of a new politically legitimate role and the defence of the professional characteristics it had acquired during the previous decades. The medical profession has struggled to maintain its jurisdictional domain, that is to say, to maintain control over the design of the health care organization and to remain as the main health actor. The objective has been to maintain health care in the professional domain. The other main confrontation with the government has to do with the characteristics of professional work and professional status. Intrinsic to its objective to maintain professional autonomy, the profession has fought to prevent bureaucratization of its work organization and practice. It has also confronted the government to maintain the possibilities of liberal practice and to prevent the proletarianization of new groups of physicians. Its objective has not only been to maintain its autonomy but also to keep its members' special status as professionals, not as civil servants or workers, within the public system.

The profession is not a monolithic community and we should note the existence of a major split in values and political projects. The strongest organizations are at the moment the most conservative ones: the Official Medical Association and the *Confederación Española de Sindicatos Médicos* (the main professional union). They acknowledge the benefits that the leading role of the state offers the profession but, while advocating the financial responsibility of the state over health care and the maintenance of an extensive public system, support the strengthening of the private market. They are the strongest supporters of a special professional status for physicians working in the public system and their objective is to save as many of the features associated with a liberal status as possible. Over the years dissident voices within the profession have become stronger and a set of radical organizations have entered into its political dynamics, challenging the dominant ideology and representational role of conservative organizations. *Federación de Asociaciones para la Defensa de la Sanidad Pública* (the left-wing political organization of professional interests) and the traditional labour unions the *Comisiones Oberas* and the *Unión General de Trabajadores* are very strong supporters of the role of the state and advocate the extension of the public system to the limit of excluding the private system. They tend to see physicians as (educated) labour, and in their language as *'trabajadores de la salud'* (health workers), but not as independent professionals. As a result they support the regulation of physicians' work and favour the end of their privileges and status within the public system. Although the strength of these organizations is not as great as that of the conservative organizations, their ties to the (external) political system have granted them considerable political power within the profession and within the health care system. The transformation of the profession and the growing number of new physicians in salaried positions widens their potential constituency and poses a threat to the traditional dominance of 'professional' ideology.

Several factors, including the failure of the public system to deliver health care efficiently, the inability of the socialist governments to organize health care according to their principles (Lluch 1983), and the incapacity of the state to deal with growing health care costs, have led to the abandonment of the socializing reform plans of the *Partido Socialista Obrero Español* (which have been replaced by projects related to the privatization of health care) and have favoured the growth of the private market. The 'failure' of the public sector has been forcing the administration to yield increasing parts of the health care market to private initiatives (de Pablo 1991). The complexity (in size, tasks and financing) of the current health care system precludes individual physicians from entering the private market as independent practitioners while thrusting the role on to large financial corporations in the health insurance and health care provision markets. The traditional influence (domain) of the profession over the private market is beginning to be threatened by the entrance of such large corporations (not controlled by physicians) into the health care business.

The 'corporatization' of medicine, accelerated with the privatizing plans of the socialist administration since 1990, further threaten the profession's 'project of survival'. The public sector, where the profession kept a great deal of control and was able to maintain 'loose' and not very bureaucratized work relations, is now subject to 'rationalization' as well as in stagnation. And its share of the private market is starting to shrink in the face of the growing share of large corporations. It seems as though a growing number of physicians are going to be forced into salaried employments and relations and into bureaucratization, without much liberal practice to compensate for their loss in control and autonomy. In consequence, large sectors of the profession (including the most conservative ones) and their organizations defended the maintenance of the public domain over health care even more than the administration when the public/private debate arose again at the beginning of the 1990s (El Pais, 27 July 1991). Within the public system the profession is still able to keep some kind of 'professional' status, exert some influence over the organization of its work and its practice, and professional criteria still have some leverage on the design and objectives of the health care system. The profession's fascination with the private market sensibly diminished when it realized that work conditions within large and complex private organizations might be closer to pure 'salaried' positions than work within publicly run organizations, normally with high levels of organizational autonomy. Curiously, it seems as though the survival of some of its 'liberal-profession' features depends on the strength of the public sector rather than on the private sector.

THE FUTURE OF THE PROFESSION

The development of the Spanish medical profession during the past five decades has been closely tied to the construction of the public health care system. The state has been the main protagonist in the construction of the medical market and as a result it has had a crucial input in the shaping of the profession itself. The profession has also had an important role both in the ideological definition of the system and in the shaping of the health care structure. As we have seen, the profession benefits enormously from the state's initiative. It has undergone spectacular growth and has also been able to build a professional practice where it combines bureaucratized work in complex organizations with types of practice very close to the liberal model. The state becomes the main sponsor of the profession both in terms of ownership of the organization where it practises medicine and in terms of the market. To a large extent, the state, as the main health insurance and health care provider, controls health demand (Derber 1982). The control of the profession over the demand for its services is small and is restricted to those areas of the market where there is private and individual practice.

The movement of health care systems towards complex health organizations has sensibly reduced the power of the profession in the organization of its work as employee. In the case of the Spanish medical profession this process has speeded up since the beginning of the 1980s with the acute financial crisis of the state and the 'need' to impose 'rational productive criteria' in public health organizations. The profession is losing little by little the 'bureaucratic' and 'production' control of these organizations. The increase in the costs of organization of medical work and the difficulties of articulating its own demand facilitates the appearance of private complex organizations (where the professional has very little control) which further limits the development of individual practice. Although some important health care insurance companies and health care organizations have been created during the past decades, and are controlled by cooperatives of physicians and directly by the Official Medical Association[3] (mostly to cover the failure of the public system in primary health care), the financial scope of the current health care organization hinders the attempts of physicians to create an alternative health care structure.

With the state's curtailment of the public system's expansion at the beginning of the 1990s and its facilitation of private sector growth, it seems clear that the Spanish medical profession is not going to be the protagonist of the new health system. Given the dimensions of the health care market and industry, large corporations are likely to take over the dominant role in the development of the private health sector. In this new framework the profession is probably closer to 'proletarianization' than within the public domain. The liberalization of the Spanish care system started by the socialist administration (from 1990 onwards) will provide clear benefits to the health corporations but might also mean the end of the individual practice the profession was able to develop during the expansion and dominance of the public system. Ultimately, this may depend on the profession's capacity to negotiate its role with the new emerging private corporations and on its political participation in the development of the new private health market.

The increasing tendency to bureaucratization and rationalization of public organizations is even threatening the technical control and autonomy of the profession. If its professional criteria (service orientation) are dominant in the public sector, the profession's level of technical autonomy will be high; but if the productivity rationality criteria become dominant (and the profession loses ideological power in the definition of the objectives of the organization of the system), then its autonomy will be severely reduced.

It seems as though the Spanish medical profession is now at another historical crossroads. It has adapted well to the parameters of development of the health system during past decades and now these parameters are changing. The great challenge to the profession during the 1990s will be to stand against the forces that lead it to bureaucratization and salarization, and to prevent the 'proletarianization' of more members and parts of the profession.

The medical profession enters the 1990s facing new challenges. A new political scenario has been built. The profession has lost its corporatist relationship with the state, there is an important fragmentation of interests and representation, and it has not yet been able to construct a mechanism for stable political participation. Not only that, but its power in health care policy-making has diminished with the increasing role of government regulators as well as large financial interests. During the 1980s a new health market and a whole new set of health care interests emerged. Public medicine and individual independent practice shrank while salaried employment increased. Profit-making is accepted as part of the new ideology of privatization, seen as the only means of putting health care back into shape, and has started replacing the idea of serving and satisfying the needs of the public, which are central to the 'professional' ideology and project. The substitution of service by profit would transform professional parameters as much as it would replace professional control over health care by managerial control. The transformation of the health care market parameters (the change in public and private roles) poses a new political challenge to the profession. Its political organizations were mainly created to deal (quite successfully) with the state but lack any experience, project and political tools to deal with the new health care system and its interests. To a large extent its political survival will depend on its capacity to create a new project of professional growth (or survival) adequate to the new market, its ability to create (or adapt existing) organizations capable of entering into the new political dynamics, and its efficiency in designing its political strategy taking into account the new distribution of forces within health care.

NOTES

1   The *Instituto Nacional de la Salud* is Social Security's health care administration and organization.
2   The *Seguro Obligatorio de Enfermedad* was the Compulsory Public Health Care Insurance the Franco regime created in 1942 as the first step towards the construction of its public health care system.
3   Four of the ten top health care insurance companies of the country (which gather 65 per cent of all premiums) are linked to the Official Medical Association, and the second one (ASISA) is owned by a cooperative of physicians.

REFERENCES

Centro de Investigaciones Sociológicas (1983) *Encuesta Nacional a los Médicos Españoles*.
Derber, C. (ed.) (1982) *Professionals as Workers: Mental Labor in Advanced Capitalism*, Boston: G. K. Hall.
Guillén, M. F. (1987) 'Procesos de cambio en la estructura ocupativa del sector sanitario español', *Revista Española de Investigaciones Sociológicas* 37: 137–204.
Instituto de Estudios de la Seguridad Social (1979) *Encuestas Nacionales a Médicos, Farmacéuticos, Veterinarios, ATS, y Público en General Sobre la Organización Sanitaria Española y Su Posible Reforma*, Madrid: IESS.
Linz, J., Orizo, F. and Gómez Reino, M. (1982) *Informe Sociológico Sobre el Cambio Político en España 1975–1981*, Madrid: FOESSA.
Lluch, E. (1983) *Política General del Ministerio de Sanidad y Consumo*, Madrid: MSC.
Mansilla, P. P. (1986) *Reforma Sanitaria: Fundamentos para un Análisis*, Madrid: MSC.
Maravall, J. M. (1982) *La Política de la Transición*, Madrid: Taurus.
Martín López, E. (1979) 'Los médicos españoles y su ideología profesional', *Revista de Seguridad Social* 2: 167–215.
de Miguel, J. M. (1976) *La Reforma Sanitaria en España*, Madrid: Cambio 16.
—— (1979) *La Sociedad Enferma*, Madrid: Akal.
de Miguel, J. M. and Guillén, M. F. (1987) 'The case of Spain', in M. G. Field (ed.), *Cross National Studies of Health Care Systems*, London: Tavistock.
Ministerio de Sanidad y Consumo (1984) *La Reforma Sanitaria a Debate, Desdeuna Perspectiva Nacional e Internacional*, Madrid: MSC.
Nadal, J. (1984) *Oferta y Demanda de Médicos en España*, Madrid: Ministerio de Sanidad y Consumo.
Organización Médica Colegial (1985) *Dos Años de Relaciones con la Administración: Informes, Propuestas y Documentos Alternativos a los Proyectos Normativos del Gobierno*, Madrid: Consejo General de Colegios Oficiales de Médicos.
Ortún, V. and Segura, A. (1983) 'España: democracia, crisis económica y política sanitaria', *Revista de Sanidad e Higiene Pública* 57: 67–89.
de Pablo, F. L. (1991) 'García Valverde expuso en el Parlamento su programa sanitario', *Tribuna Médica* May: 3–5.
Pérez Díaz, V. (1982) 'Médicos, administradores y enfermos', *Papeles de Economía Española* 12–13: 231–51.
Rodríguez, J. A. (1987) *Salud y Sociedad*, Madrid: Tecnos.
—— (1990) 'Political dynamics of physician manpower policy: the case of Spain', *Health Policy* 15: 119–42.
—— (1992) 'Struggle and revolt: the changing role of the Spanish medical profession', *International Journal of Health Services* 22(1): 19–44.
Saturno, P. (1987) 'The health care system in Spain: on a wave of change', in R. Saltman (ed.), *International Handbook of Health Care Systems*, London: Greenwood.

Schmitter, P. and Lehmbruch, G. (eds) (1979) *Trends in Corporatist Intermediation*, Beverly Hills: Sage.

Servicio de Estudios Sociológicos del Instituto de Estudios de la Seguridad Social (1979) 'Encuesta nacional sobre la organización sanitaria y su posible reforma', *Revista de Seguridad Social* 3: 259–93.

10 The Belgian medical profession since the 1980s

Dominance and decline?

Rita Schepers

Since the 1980s the Belgian medical profession has come under increased pressures. These are primarily related to its position within the Health Insurance System and *vis-à-vis* the sickness funds. Whether these developments amount to professional decline and erosion of professional autonomy is not yet clear. For several reasons caution is required. First of all, most policy changes are recent and it is hard to predict what consequences their implementation will have for the medical profession, not in the least because there is little or no systematic information available. In other instances, we are only talking of proposals. Second, the significance of these developments can only be understood if account is taken of the previous history of the medical profession, especially in its relationship with the Health Insurance System and the sickness funds. But even a long-term perspective does not provide clear answers as to the direction of change in professional status. One has to decide which points in history are the basis for comparison. As will be illustrated, certain policy changes were unthinkable a decade ago and certain proposals which seem to be considered seriously today encountered fierce opposition in the 1960s. But it is doubtful whether compared to the pre-Second World War situation the autonomy of the profession is declining. Third, even the contrast of the present and the recent past does not give enough evidence to draw any firm conclusions with respect to the nature of the changes in the social position of Belgian physicians, because it is not clear how far changes have to go before one can speak of a diminution of autonomy. Moreover, not all segments of the profession seem to be affected by the changes to the same extent. Last but not least, what we are witnessing is a process of change in the Health Insurance System as a whole, affecting the position of all participants. Since the postwar position of the medical profession is closely related to that of the Health Insurance System, its position is also changing, but not necessarily declining.

In this chapter, the following points will be addressed. The first section will describe the general features of the social position of the Belgian medical profession, with emphasis on its relationship with the Health Insurance System, and give a brief overview of the relationship between the two main parties in the Belgian health care field in this century: the sickness funds and the medical profession. Needless to say, a comprehensive account of decades of development cannot be presented here. The second section focuses on the changing position of physicians since the 1980s. The final section will draw some conclusions.

THE BELGIAN MEDICAL PROFESSION AND THE HEALTH INSURANCE SYSTEM PRIOR TO THE 1980s

The autonomy of the Belgian profession in the Health Insurance System

Following Elston (1991: 61–2), one can distinguish between technical, economic and political autonomy. Economic autonomy is defined as the right of doctors to determine their remuneration; political autonomy as the right of doctors to make policy decisions as the legitimate experts on health matters; and clinical or technical autonomy as the right of the profession to set its own standards and control clinical performance, exercised, for example, through clinical freedom at the bedside, professional control over recruitment and training or collegial control over discipline and malpractice.

Medicine in Belgium offers a good example of a profession with a clear, legal monopoly over medical practice, considerable political, economic and clinical autonomy and a position of dominance within the health care field. Its legal position has been shaped by three laws enacted in the 1960s, in Belgium the golden era of doctoring: the Law on Health and Disability Insurance of 1963, complemented by the Agreement of 25 June 1964, the Royal Decree No. 78 on the Practice of Medicine and the Royal Decree No. 79 on the Order of Physicians, both dating from 1967. First, the most relevant aspects of these legal acts will be discussed in chronological order. Second, the Belgian profession, and in particular the two most influential medical syndicates, will be introduced.

By the Law of 28 December 1944, social security was established in Belgium. The Regent's Decree of 21 March 1945, in implementation of article 6 of the Law of 1944, introduced compulsory health and disability insurance for all wage-earners (about 60 per cent of the population). The existing sickness funds, while remaining private organizations, were charged with the administration of health and disability insurance. The doctors' organization at that time, the *Fédération Médicale Belge*, refused any kind of agreement within the framework of the new law. In practice, this meant that the system of direct payment of the physician by the patient – which was strongly advocated by the *Fédération Médicale Belge* before the war – was maintained. Every practitioner, according to what was known as the 'direct agreement principle', remained free to set his or her fee for each patient (albeit that they were urged to respect the minimum fee levels established by their professional organization). The sickness funds reimbursed a set percentage of the physician's fee (which should have been 75 per cent for general practice and 100 per cent for specialist care). But since national negotiations between sickness funds and medical profession about fee-schedules were absent, the sickness funds unilaterally decided on the level of the fees – always lower than the actual fee charged by physicians – and their reimbursement. Whenever sickness funds tried to bridge the gap by raising their (theoretical) fees and reimbursement, doctors reacted by raising the actual fee and the gap was maintained (Dejardin 1991: 78).

From the beginning, the Health Insurance System had been afflicted by several problems. Not only did the medical profession cause difficulties, but also the relationship between the major sickness funds was strained and, moreover, the financial situation of the Health Insurance System was bleak. The government attempted to remedy this situation at the beginning of the 1960s with a fundamental review of the Health Insurance System. One of the aims of the reform was the introduction of a 'negotiated agreement' in order to establish medical fees by periodic collective negotiation. In the preliminary negotiations, the leaders of the professional organizations at that time were willing to share responsibility and cooperate by means of agreements with the Health Insurance System on condition that the so-called principles of the medical charter would be respected. These principles are: unrestricted free choice of a doctor by the patient, the safeguarding of medical confidentiality and professional independence, which means control of doctors by their colleagues. However, the leadership was overridden by a more militant membership, which declined to take any financial responsibility for the Health Insurance System. Indeed, according to this medical opposition, to share financial responsibility was nothing less than agreeing to the rationing of medical care, and this would harm patients. The crisis led to the demise of the *Fédération Médicale Belge* and the birth of medical syndicates. The *Fédération Nationale des Chambres Syndicales des Médecins* (National Federation of Syndicalist Chambers of Doctors), better known, after the name of its first secretary-general, as the Wynen syndicate, established in 1962, has dominated medical syndicalism since then.

In the light of present changes, it is good to remember what was at stake at the beginning of the 1960s. The following five issues were of particular importance. First, as has already been explained, in Belgium a reimbursement system prevailed. In the original proposals for reform by the government, reimbursement by the sickness fund would be lower when a doctor refused to cooperate with the Health Insurance System. This 'discrimination' between doctors was alleged to undermine the free choice of the doctor by the patient. Second, sanctions for not respecting the agreed fee-schedules could take the form of imprisonment. This measure would undermine professional honour and dignity. Third, in order to promote the cost-effectiveness as well as the quality of medical care, the government wanted physicians to keep records of the care provided (*'un carnet de prestation'*). Information could be requested by the medical inspectors of the sickness funds and the *Institut National d'Assurance Maladie-Invalidité* (National Institute for Sickness and Invalidity Insurance). But this proposal was considered to threaten medical confidentiality. Fourth, article 35 of the proposed Law on Health and Disability Insurance stipulated that care had to be delivered to the insured in the most economical way compatible with the preservation and the improvement of their health. According to the medical opposition, this constituted an infringement on the freedom of therapy of physicians and introduced non-medical criteria in the delivery of medical care. Last but not least, although shared responsibility was rejected – a doctor's place was at the side of his or her patients – doctors were willing to participate in the activities of a technical medical council, on the condition that it would be exclusively composed of physicians and dependent only on the medical profession. Looking at the arguments used, it is striking that professional ethics – at least a liberal version of them – played a crucial role in defending the autonomy of the medical profession.

Mainly under pressure of the Wynen syndicate, the government agreed to modify the Law on Health and Disability Insurance accepted by Parliament on 9 August 1963 in order to take into account the desiderata of the dominant medical syndicate (Law of 24 December 1963). Despite this conciliatory stance, the dominant medical syndicate called a strike in 1964, in order to demonstrate its power and willingness to use that power. The strike was justified as being for the benefit of the patient. In the perception of the syndicate, good medical care, responsive to the needs of the patient, is linked to the independence of the medical profession.

The profession's position within the Health Insurance System was established after an eighteen-day strike resulting in important concessions from the government. With the agreement of 25 June 1964 (also called the St John's agreement) its autonomy and influence within the Health Insurance System was established. First, at its own request, the medical profession was only to be represented within the General Council and the Board of Directors of the Office for Medical Care within the *Institut National d'Assurance Maladie-Invalidité* in an advisory role. However, it accepted equal numerical representation with that of the sickness funds within powerful committees, such as the Committee for Medical Control, the Technical Medical Council and the National Commission of Doctors and Sickness Funds. The Technical Medical Council is composed exclusively of doctors, appointed by the sickness funds, by the representative organizations of the medical profession and by the medical faculties. The Technical Medical Council is responsible for establishing the 'nomenclature' – a relative value scale for a list of medical acts grouped under a number of 'key letters'. With its decision as to which technical acts with which relative weight should be considered for reimbursement, the Technical Medical Council had (and still has) a profound impact on medical practice. The monetary multipliers for the 'key letters' are decided in the National Commission of Doctors and Sickness Funds (*Commission Médico-Mutualiste*).

These commissions are important channels to influence the policies of the Health Insurance System in directions favourable to the interests of the profession. And it is the Health Insurance System which determines to a very great extent health care policy in Belgium. 'Health-care policy and decision-making processes are captured within an overall framework of costs, expenditures and financing' (Nuyens 1986: 225). Second, the principles of the medical charter – in other words liberal medical ideology – were incorporated within the insurance system. Freedom of choice of the physician by the patient, medical confidentiality and diagnostic and therapeutic freedom were guaranteed. With respect to the latter issue, the revised article 35 stipulated that physicians decide in full freedom and according to their conscience about the care to be delivered to patients. Abuses would be controlled by the Order of Physicians (see later). It was the most liberal regulation within the then six countries of the European Economic Community (van Langendonck 1971: 213). In other issues related to professional ethics, too, the position of the Order was reinforced. Third, national agreements were to be concluded between the medical profession and the sickness funds and to be approved by the government. Doctors were absolutely free to accept these agreements. For those who accepted them, deviations from the fee-schedule were allowed for home calls or weekend services and at certain times during each week (not to exceed 25 per cent of working hours). Doctors who decided to remain outside the Health Insurance System could charge any fee they liked, but the patient could obtain reimbursement only for 75 per cent of the official fee. The government accepted that only in those regions of Belgium where 60 per cent or more of all doctors (50 per cent of the general practitioners and 50 per cent of the specialists) agreed to the negotiated fee-schedule did it have to be followed. In the absence of an agreement, the government could impose fees or fix the reimbursement levels. One inducement for doctors to observe fees was a policy of the *Institut National d'Assurance Maladie-Invalidité* to make an annual contribution to a retirement fund for each doctor who agreed to abide by the schedule. After 1964, the government still had few instruments to influence or monitor the behaviour of physicians.

The two Royal Decrees of 1967 were enacted without any parliamentary debate under a government with special powers. It has been suggested that this remarkable procedure was related to the leading politicians' judgement that the political costs of tangling with competing medical syndicates were too high (Dillemans 1974: 175). The position of autonomy of the medical profession was reinforced by the Royal Decree No. 78 of 1967 on the Practice of Medicine, also called the Law on the Practice of Medicine. This law confirmed first of all the legal monopoly over medical practice of the 'doctor of medicine, surgery and obstetrics'. The monopoly is far-reaching and covers every aspect of medicine, including alternative medicine. With the exception of France, Belgium is probably the only Western European country where the legal position of physicians has been regulated in detail by the legislature (Nys and Quaethoven 1984: 57). For example, the Royal Decree of 1967 specifies the right to diagnostic and therapeutic freedom, the safeguarding of medical confidentiality and the right to fees or salaries in accordance with the principles of the code of ethics. It contains a number of prescriptions that in other countries are part of medical ethics, such as the prohibition of fee-splitting and of the abuse of diagnostic and therapeutic freedom. Last but not least, the control over key issues of medical practice lies in the hands of the Order of Physicians.

The Order had been established in 1938, but was reorganized in 1967 (Schepers 1979: 130). This reorganization has significantly enlarged the Order's jurisdiction in particular over faults committed outside the professional sphere of activities. The Order of Physicians is a state-sanctioned, disciplinary council of which membership is compulsory for all practising physicians. Its sanctions are powerful, since disenrolment bans a physician from practice. The Order's disciplinary boards – ten Provincial Councils and two Councils of Appeal – are composed of physicians, elected by their colleagues, and of magistrates. Medical syndicates lobby strongly to have their members elected into the (Provincial) Councils of the Order. The National Council of the Order received in 1967 the power to formulate a code of medical ethics. The draft code produced in 1975 reflected the liberal ideology of the dominant groups within the medical profession. Because of severe criticism from several important groups in the health care field, such as the sickness funds, but also from within the profession, the code has not yet received approval by Royal Decree. However, the Belgian Supreme Court has accepted the binding force of several articles of the draft (Nys and Quaethoven 1984: 58). The Law on the Practice of Medicine and the Law on the Order of Physicians incorporates a liberal model of medicine and imposes it not only on all medical practitioners, but also on other health care providers. This is one aspect of the medical dominance of the Belgian profession. The position of nursing and of the paramedical occupations is clearly subordinate to medicine. Nursing obtained protection of its domain in 1974, but the implementation of major aspects of this law was delayed until 1990. Paramedical occupations only obtained protection of title in 1990. In 1993 a review of the Law on the Practice of Medicine was announced.

Although its legal position is quite strong, the Belgian medical profession lacks one instrument for the safeguarding of its autonomy, that is, control over the number of entrants to the profession. The reasons for refusing this are manifold. The fear of reinforcing the already considerable power and dominance of the profession, linked with the refusal to grant a staunchly liberal profession this form of market closure, certainly played an important role.

Finally, the professional organization of physicians needs some attention. Clearly, the profession does not speak with one voice. First, there is a structural differentiation between medical faculties, medical syndicates, scientific organizations, the Order of Physicians, the Royal Academy of Medicine and so on. Suffice it to say that their interests are not always, or, even more accurately, often not, identical. The two major medical syndicates are the *Belgische Vereniging van Artsensyndikaten* (Belgian Association of Medical Syndicates[1]) and the *Algemeen Syndikaat der Geneesheren van België* (General Syndicate of Belgian Physicians), respectively known as the Wynen syndicate and the De Brabanter syndicate. The first organization claims to speak in the name of the majority of the Belgian physicians. The two syndicates represent different models of medical practice. The *Belgische Vereniging van Artsensyndikaten* defends 'liberal medicine' in its classic form, characterized by great autonomy and dominance in the health care field. The *Algemeen Syndikaat der Geneesheren van België*, which is more moderate, is prepared to cooperate with and share responsibility for the Health Insurance System. In order to comply with criteria for representation of doctors in official committees within the *Institut National d'Assurance Maladie-Invalidité*, the *Algemeen Syndikaat der Geneesheren van België* formed in 1975 a coalition – the Confederation of Belgian Physicians – with two smaller groups: a regional group of doctors which separated from Wynen and a group of general practitioners. The *Belgische Vereniging van Artsensyndikaten* and the Confederation represent doctors in negotiations, for example on fee schedules within the *Institut National d'Assurance Maladie-Invalidité*. Of the eleven medical representatives in the important National Commission of Doctors and Sickness Funds, nine are members of the Wynen syndicate and two represent the Confederation. However, the relative strength of these organizations is unknown and in the past plans to hold elections to determine exactly how strong they are were rejected by Wynen. Apart from these divisions, there is opposition between general practitioners and specialists, between Flemings and Walloons, between younger and older doctors, and personal hostilities are rife. Only when seriously threatened do ranks close against the enemy.

The medical profession and the sickness funds

Essential to the understanding of the current shape of the Belgian health care system is the fact that it is the outcome of a struggle not only between the medical profession and the sickness funds, but also between two conflicting ideologies on health insurance: the Christian and the socialist (Pasture 1992: 144). From the beginning, the Belgian Health Insurance System relied on private sickness funds which were grouped along denominational/political lines. This was part of the pillarization of Belgian society. 'A "pillar" as a sociological concept is a set of closed, tightly interlocking organizations held together by a common cultural orientation' (Therborn 1989: 202). Catholics and socialists, who form the two most important 'pillars', differed with respect to their views on the most desirable organization not only of the Health Insurance System, but also of the health care system. Catholics defended institutional pluralism with the government in a subsidiary role. The early sickness funds were considered to be self-help organizations. Later the accent shifted towards funds as insurance companies. In both cases, strong emphasis was laid on the responsibility of the members for the efficient organization of their fund. On this view, sickness funds should carry financial responsibility. With respect to the organization of health care, Catholics were in favour of private initiative with government support if required (*liberté subsidiée*). The socialists, on the other hand, favoured the establishment of apolitical, regional, unitary sickness funds. In their view it was the task of the state to develop a social security system for all its citizens. It was also the state which had to carry financial responsibility for the system. With respect to the organization of health care more emphasis was placed on the role of public institutions. Moreover, a systematic organization of health care with a clear division between primary, secondary and tertiary care was advocated. To simplify, one could argue that within Belgium, advocates of a Bismarckian Health Insurance System and a kind of National Health Service were represented by ideologically opposed groupings with comparable strength.

The idea of a unified insurance structure appealed to the *Fédération Médicale*

Belge, but it was hostile to most other ideas emanating from the Socialist Party and sickness funds. The Catholic Party and the Christian sickness funds with their emphasis on private initiative, self-regulation and autonomy were in general more sympathetic to the profession's claims, but of course rejected the latter's insistence on the abolition of the so-called 'political' sickness funds. After the First World War, the role of the sickness funds in health care policy became gradually more important (Schepers 1993a: 385). This expansion came about without any consultation with the leadership of the *Fédération Médicale Belge*, which caused great resentment among a very large sector of the profession. Probably under influence of this development, the *Fédération Médicale Belge* increasingly favoured solo practice, with payments on a fee-for-service basis, to individual clients with little or no external control over decision-making. The organization seems to have been successful in imposing its viewpoint on the sickness funds, mainly by making cooperation dependent on the acceptance of certain conditions which together form the medical charter. In the 1920s, the institutional structure, characteristic of the relationship between sickness funds and medical profession within the Health Insurance System, began to be developed with the establishment of joint commissions of representatives of sickness funds and the *Fédération Médicale Belge* ('*commission médico-mutualiste*') mainly to negotiate fee levels. Last but not least, in the face of mounting criticisms by the sickness funds of the rising costs of medical and pharmaceutical services and the poor quality of medical services, the campaign for the establishment of an Order of Physicians intensified in the 1920s. The Order had to regulate the profession in the public interest. But at the same time the *Fédération Médicale Belge* considered the Order as an instrument to assist its efforts to promote solo fee-for-service practice (Schepers 1993a: 388). Although the medical profession was faced with what it considered to be the great political and economic strength of the sickness funds, the latter's ideological divisions weakened the threat to the medical profession. The system, which was highly competitive, was dogged by financial problems, which intensified the strain on the relationship between sickness funds and medical practitioners.

As was described earlier, opposition to the involvement of politically dominated groups in the health care system continued after the Second World War. The medical profession has continued to criticize the role assumed by the sickness funds in health care policy. In its opinion, sickness funds are mere counters to pay insurance monies to the insured and can easily be disposed of.

It needs to be emphasized that the autonomy of the sickness funds matches that of the medical profession. Until 1990, sickness funds were regulated by an out-dated law of 1894. The Law of 1963 introduced financial responsibility for the sickness funds. But this regulation has never been put into practice. Since 1964, physicians together with sickness funds have played a dominant role in directing the policies of the Health Insurance System. Some observers speak of a '*Pax Medica*' (Medical Peace) to draw attention to the fact that doctors and sickness funds agreed tacitly in the 1960s to slice up the national cake, which the government, employers and employees are paying for, and to avoid fundamental conflicts, which could threaten the '*Pax Medica*' that after all was rewarding for both parties (see, for example, Nuyens 1985: 32). Both are represented in equal strength within important commissions within the Health Insurance System. Both sides have expertise and power, albeit of a different kind. The government and the social partners (employers and trade unions) who are also supposed to carry responsibility for the Health Insurance System are, in fact, less influential. As neither sickness funds nor physicians took any financial responsibility for the Health Insurance System, it is not surprising that this open-ended public expenditure commitment resulted in huge budgetary deficits.

DEVELOPMENTS SINCE THE 1980s

The medical profession and the Health Insurance System

The themes of policy-making throughout the decade are related to the financial difficulties of the Health Insurance System and the responsibility of the two main actors in it – the medical profession and sickness funds – for the present situation. The new law on the sickness funds (1990) and the Health Insurance System (1993), the bill on reform of the Order of Physicians (1989) and the development of instruments to control the efficiency with which resources are used share the objective of enhancing the cost-effectiveness of the system. They illustrate not only the preoccupation of the government with cost-containment, but also its greater determination to push its policy through. Second, the determination to take on the medical profession could be linked to the perceived weakness of the profession, which is partly due to the growing number of physicians and the increased competition between individual practitioners, but also to the intense rivalry between often small, but always vociferous, professional associations. If this was the case, the profession proved more resilient then expected. Third, the absence of any fundamental change with respect to the position of the medical profession and the Health Insurance System as a whole could be linked to the gridlock between sickness funds – once again divided over the issue of financial accountability – and even more important between Wallony and Flanders with respect to an eventual federalization of the Health Insurance System (Schepers 1993b).

Financial difficulties as well as acrimonious relations between the sickness funds and the medical profession have beset the Health Insurance System from the beginning and in this respect the 1980s were no different from previous decades. However, they differed in the ferocity of the confrontation. In the 1980s, concern over escalating costs led to growing financial constraints. The government – from 1982 until 1988 a coalition of Christian-Democrats and Liberals – had a strong commitment to reducing public expenditure. Probably partly as a result of this, a slump occurred in the relations between the sickness funds and the medical profession. In 1983 the dominant medical syndicate filed a complaint against the sickness funds. In 1987 a judicial inquiry into the sickness funds revealed the existence of fraud, misappropriation of funds (an estimated 2.3 billion BF between 1979 and 1982), forgery and fraudulous accounting. Even though the verdict of the court in 1991 cleared the sickness funds of most charges, their legitimacy had been seriously affected. As if to maintain the equilibrium, figures about the number of doctors deviating from the official fee were published by the *Institut National d'Assurance Maladie-Invalidité*. Although there was long-standing evidence that improper charges were levied, fees until the 1980s were rarely challenged. Now the sickness funds and the mass media attacked specialists – among whom deviations are believed to be greater than among general practitioners – for charging excessively high fees. These events demonstrated first the extent to which the sickness funds and the medical profession alike had been living off the Health Insurance System. Second, it became clear that the government did not have an adequate grip on how money was used by the sickness funds nor by the medical profession. As a reaction to the so-called sickness fund scandal, plans to reform not only the sickness funds and the Health Insurance System but also – and significantly – the Order of Physicians were unveiled. First the measures related to the sickness funds and the Health Insurance System will briefly be discussed. Then the focus will again be turned on the medical profession.

In 1990 a new Law on the sickness funds was enacted replacing the obsolete Law of 1894. For the purpose of this analysis, the following points are of importance. In general the sickness funds preserved their central role in health care policy. Legally they can deploy activities related to the improvement of the health of their members. Health is defined in terms of the World Health Organization definition as 'a state of physical, mental and social well-being'. Apart from strengthening independent financial control over the sickness funds and creating greater structural clarity, their democratic character was reinforced, hence legitimating their claim of being representatives of the consumers. Moreover, the sickness funds received the legal right to represent their members in court in cases of doctors overcharging patients. Of course, this caused outrage from the medical profession, which considered it as an instrument to pressurize and blackmail doctors.

In the Programme-laws of 1991 and 1992 a global budget for health care expenditure and separate budgets for certain sectors, such as radiology, clinical biology, medicines and hospital care, were introduced, and correction mechanisms were devised for when the budgets would be exceeded. In 1993, a new law on health and disability insurance (Law Moureaux) was accepted by Parliament. Without going into detail, the following points need to be mentioned. First, the hands of the financiers of the Health Insurance System – employers, trade unions and government – were strengthened. They were made responsible for the setting of a global budget for health care expenditure and separate budgets for specific sectors. Initially, the medical profession as well as the sickness funds were pushed to the background in the matter of deciding how the budget would be divided. Following strong opposition by the (Christian) funds, sickness funds obtained representation within the General Management Board of the Health

Insurance System and the General Council of the Office for Medical Care in a decision-making capacity. Doctors are not represented within the first body and within the second they remain, as before, in an advisory role. Second, the activities of agreement and convention commissions are supervised by an Insurance Committee (comparable to the former Board of Directors) in which sickness funds have a dominant role. Third, in the agreement commissions, such as the Commission of Doctors and Sickness Funds, doctors and sickness funds are equally represented. A budget control commission is charged with the supervision of the achievement of budgetary targets and with the task of proposing adjustments to them. Medical syndicates are in a minority position here. The Minister would have the power to intervene if health care providers and sickness funds do not succeed in meeting their budgetary targets.

The plan to set budgets for all sectors of medical practice, the power of the Minister to intervene unilaterally in agreements when budgetary targets are not met, as well as other government proposals related to the third-party payer system and specialist medical fees in hospitals led the Wynen syndicate to campaign not to renew the agreement between the Health Insurance System and doctors in 1993. This campaign proved successful (51.5 per cent of physicians rejected the government proposal although with different results in Flanders compared to Wallony and among general practitioners compared to specialists). As a result, for the first time since 1964, there is no negotiated agreement and medical fees are, in theory, free of restriction. In practice, the majority of doctors seem to abide by the fees proposed by the Minister. The point they wanted to make was one of principle, that is, to reject what they considered to be an attack on liberal medicine. In subsequent negotiations with the Wynen syndicate, it seems that the government was willing to concede a number of points. Specific budgets will only be set for the four sectors mentioned above. Moreover, the Minister promised measures to limit the number of entrants to medical faculties in the future. Furthermore, money will be collected for the health care sector by raising the co-payment charges.

As mentioned before, following the sickness funds scandal, the Minister of Social Affairs also intended to change the organization of the Order of Physicians. The social function as well as the composition of the Order were to be changed. The new-style Order had to maintain and improve the quality of medical care in the interest of the patient and to take into account the limited resources available for its provision. Apart from dedication, expertise, tact, delicacy and integrity, doctors were also expected to behave with moderation and responsibility with respect to the basic principles of solidarity, embodied in and essential to every system of social security. Therefore the Order had to monitor and sanction violations of the law related to diagnostic and therapeutic freedom (article 35 of the Law of 1963). To facilitate this, the obligatory advice of a medical administrator from the *Institut National d'Assurance Maladie-Invalidité* was introduced for the Provincial Councils and for the Councils of Appeal. The proposed changes were significant, first because they unveiled the government's preoccupation with the control of the economic behaviour of physicians and, second, because they suggested that there was insufficient political support for radical change. Despite long-standing and severe criticism of its functioning and calls for its abolition, especially from within the Socialist Party, and despite ample proof that it had failed in the past in self-regulation, in particular of the economic behaviour of physicians, the Order was preserved in its present form, that is, a body mainly composed of elected physicians. Finally, the reforms have never been introduced. The official reason was disagreement about the linguistic divisions within the Provincial Council of Brabant. But there are good reasons to believe that continuing opposition from the dominant medical syndicate, which threatened to boycott the planned reorganized Order, played a role as well. In this respect the delay could reflect the political strength of the profession.

However, other legal measures were introduced. The Programme-law of 22 December 1989 introduced changes in article 35 of the Law of 1963. On the one hand, the therapeutic freedom of physicians was reconfirmed, but on the other hand, physicians are now obliged 'to refrain from prescribing unnecessary, expensive investigations and treatment and from carrying out or having carried out unnecessary treatment at the expense of the obligatory Health Insurance System'. In other words, the government challenged the idea that clinical autonomy bestows the right to use public resources without limits. Moreover, instead of leaving control of abuses of diagnostic and therapeutic freedom exclusively in the hands of the Order, the government developed instruments to monitor the economic behaviour of physicians. For example, within the Committee for Medical Control of the *Institut National d'Assurance Maladie-Invalidité*, a watchdog committee, composed of physicians and magistrates, was established to evaluate the quantity of medical care. The aim is to determine transgressions of article 35 of the Law of 1963. Representative organizations of doctors and sickness funds nominate an equal number of physicians. It is also significant that only two physicians will represent the medical syndicates, one from each rival syndicate, thus undermining the traditional dominance of the *Belgische Vereniging van Artsensyndikaten*. The latter has protested furiously and filed a complaint with the Council of State, but without success. Statistical profiles of all services provided by a particular doctor are developed by profile-committees within the *Institut National d'Assurance Maladie-Invalidité*. Sanctions have been introduced, such as the temporary loss of *Institut National d'Assurance Maladie-Invalidité* contributions to a pension-fund, and for physicians punished by the Order, a committee for medical control or a court. The consequence of these measures could be a limitation of the physician's freedom to practise medicine according to his or her own clinical judgement. Nevertheless, such regulations are easier to enact than they are to apply and up until now practitioners have found numerous ways of avoiding attempts to restrict their activities.

By the end of the 1980s, not only the government but also the sickness funds seemed more willing to confront the medical profession. For example, the Christian sickness funds emphasized the potential of modern information technology to provide data on cost and outcome of doctors' activities. They suggested that, in the future, agreements may only be concluded between the Health

Insurance System and physicians willing to comply with certain conditions, such as the keeping of medical records. They also mentioned the possibility of individual contracts with physicians. The fact that this issue was revived could be an indication of the perceived weakness of the profession. And, finally, sickness funds are more actively engaged in developing quality assurance procedures than the medical profession.

The supply of physicians

By far the most serious threat to the position of the profession, in particular that of general practitioners, comes from the growing number of physicians. In 1991, Belgium had 36,178 qualified physicians or one doctor to 277 inhabitants (Schepens 1992: 54). The high density of physicians adversely affects income and status. The average annual income decreased in the course of the 1980s (Wouters *et al.* 1988: 165, 168). According to a comparative study of general practitioner incomes in the European Community, Belgian general practitioners are amongst the least well paid (van der Zee *et al.* 1991). Younger physicians report lower annual incomes than their older counterparts. A young general practitioner earns less than a young civil servant with a university degree. Figures about the number of mainly young doctors with small clienteles – about 25 per cent of them see less than seven patients a day – also suggest that, because of lack of experience, the quality of their medical work might be lower (Vereniging der Belgische Omnipractici 1992). Instead of full-time medical practice, some young general practitioners are forced to take on other jobs to supplement their incomes.

Until now the patterns of delivery of medical services have remained quite individualistic. First, general practitioners as well as specialists are predominantly engaged in private solo practice – according to information not yet published from the Flemish Scientific Association of General Practitioners, around 75 per cent of general practitioners still work in a solo practice. Nearly all specialists have staff appointments in hospitals, but only a small fraction do all their professional work there. Large group practices are rather exceptional. Second, there are no financial restraints against direct access of patients to specialists. The principle of free choice in an open medical market prevails. Third, the fee-for-service remains the dominant payment system. Even those specialists who are full-time in hospitals earn their incomes predominantly from individual patient fees, rather than salaries.

There is considerable difference of opinion among (general) practitioners about the measures to be taken. Significantly some proposals deviate from the traditional options for fee-for-service and an open medical market. Keywords in the debate in 1993 were subsidiarity, echelons, registration with and referral by general practitioners (de Jong and Schepers 1993). Subsidiarity in health care means that care will be provided on the level where it is most cost-effective, with the understanding that the delivery of primary care by specialists involves the ineffective use of resources. Each patient should register with a general practitioner and if necessary be referred to a specialist. Direct access to medical specialists should be financially sanctioned with reduced reimbursement. The payment of a lump sum in order to keep a medical file of each patient is a measure which deviates from the traditional fee-for-service. The introduction of a variety of modes of remuneration, which would be more adapted, for example, to prevention, is being advocated. A new and significant development is the plea for separate negotiations between general practitioner associations and the government. It has to be emphasized that in this case we are only talking of proposals and, given the unpredictable character of Belgian compromise politics, it would be hazardous to forecast the future.

CONCLUSION

The picture of the Belgian medical profession in the 1980s is clearly different from that in the 1960s. While in the 1960s the medical profession defiantly, aggressively – and successfully – pressed ahead its claims, it now finds itself in a defensive position, but it is far from beaten. In assessing its present situation it must be remembered that before 1964 there was no agreement between the Health Insurance System and the medical profession. More generally, the uncertainties facing the medical profession today no doubt match its uncertainties when the Health Insurance System was being developed in the interwar period and introduced in 1945. Belgian doctors, or, more specifically, the *Belgische Vereniging van Artsensyndikaten* and some smaller organizations, put the blame for faults with the sickness funds and the social security system. They are in a combative mood and ready to defend the 'last bastion of liberal medicine in Europe' against the reforms, introduced by a 'politicized' government and (to variable extent) supported by the 'political' sickness funds. However, doctors have predicted doom and decline throughout the century. It must also be remembered that almost all of the measures discussed in the second section of this paper date from the late 1980s and early 1990s. Therefore, it is with considerable caution that conclusions are drawn.

In general, the profession as a corporate entity still seems to retain much of its traditional power and autonomy within the Health Insurance System. Fundamental changes in the political autonomy of the profession have not yet occurred. It is important to emphasize that the profession's power is ultimately negative in character. Doctors' ability to influence decisions rests in part on the sanction they can exercise, that is, the withdrawal of services. The strike threat is regularly used by the *Belgische Vereniging van Artsensyndikaten* which dominates the negotiations with the sickness funds and the government. The inability of the profession to present a coherent view on its, and the health care system's, future does not necessarily mean that it will be weak and powerless when it comes to defending what it considers to be the essence of (liberal) medicine, as developments in 1993 illustrated. Therefore the strengthening of the position of the financiers and the sickness funds might prove to be less effective than it appears. With respect to economic autonomy, the medical syndicates, on the one hand, will have to take into account budgetary targets. Moreover, physicians have to respect cost-control measures, something they ardently refused not only in 1964, but also at the beginning of the 1980s. Furthermore they are more accountable in a financial sense for their actions. Against the background of the 1960s, it is significant that control of diagnostic and therapeutic freedom is no longer exclusively exercised by the profession. On the other hand, physicians are still in a position to influence the level of remuneration within the National Commission of Doctors and Sickness Funds. Probably more important, because the relationship with the sickness funds and the Health Insurance System is rather detached, they will be more or less immune from direct cost-control. However, on an individual level, the picture is different, at least for certain sections of the medical profession, such as general practitioners. A fee-for-service system does not in itself guarantee the freedom to obtain a satisfactory income. Partly as a result of the growing numbers of practitioners and the increased competition, the economic autonomy of the individual practitioner, especially the general practitioner, has decreased in the 1980s. Belgian physicians still enjoy a very large degree of clinical autonomy. The medical profession as such remains the only entity to define what is good medical practice. It still has the right to set its own standards and control clinical performance. The Technical Medical Council and other important commissions are exclusively composed of doctors. What is lacking is professional control over entrance to the medical profession. However, on an individual level, clinical autonomy is rather meaningless if there are no patients in the waiting room, or it could be threatened by the fact that, again as the result of overcrowding and competition, doctors are eager to follow patients' whims and wishes instead of their own professional judgement.

In summary, the developments since the 1980s certainly have symbolic value and could potentially be subversive to the traditional position of the medical profession. Their real test lies in the way they are implemented. At this stage it is impossible to predict whether medical authority will be eroded in the near future. But there is some cause for scepticism, not only because of the resistance of the medical profession, but also because of the fact that tensions between the two main sickness funds have resurfaced around the old issue of their financial responsibility. Even more important is the debate about the eventual federalization of the Health Insurance System. This could delay not only the implementation of certain measures, but also the fundamental revision of the system. In these debates, which will be crucial to the future position of the profession, its own voice is of minor importance.

NOTE

1   The Belgian Association of Medical Syndicates was established in 1981 and replaces the National Federation of Syndicalist Chambers of Physicians.

REFERENCES

Dejardin, J. (1991) 'De rol van de ziekenfondsen in de onderhandelingen met de zorgverstrekkers', in Landsbond der Christelijke Mutualiteiten, *De Mutualiteit Vandaag en Morgen: Wettelijk Kader, Opdrachten en Uitdagingen*, Antwerp: Kluwer.

Dillemans, R. (1974) 'De wetgevende besluiten betreffende de uitoefening van de geneeskunde in perspectief', *Tijdschrift voor Privaatrecht* 11: 173–209.

Elston, M. A. (1991) 'The politics of professional power: medicine in a changing health service', in J. Gabe, M. Calnan and M. Bury (eds), *The Sociology of the Health Service*, London: Routledge.

de Jong, B. and Schepers, R. (1993) 'General practitioners in Belgium and the Netherlands: recent developments', paper presented at conference on 'Facing the European Challenge: The Role of Professions in a Wider Europe', Leeds, 13–15 July.

Kesenne, K., Hermesse, J. and Soete, R. (1991) 'Financiële verantwoordelijkheid: een regeling voor de toekomst', in Landsbond der Christelijke Mutualiteiten, *De Mutualiteit Vandaag en Morgen: Wettelijk Kader, Opdrachten en Uitdagingen*, Antwerp: Kluwer.

van Langendonck, J. (1971) *De Harmonisering van de Sociale Verzekering voor Gezondheidszorgen in de EEG*, Leuven: University Press.

Marchal, O. (1989) *Où allez-vous Dr Wynen? Le patron des médecins Belges répond à O. Marchal*, Brussels: Didier Hatier.

Nuyens, Y. (1985) 'Knelpunten in de gezondheidszorg', in H. Nys, M. Foets and J. Mertens (eds), *Organisatie van de Gezondheidszorg in Vlaanderen*, Antwerp: Van Loghum Slaterus.

—— (1986) 'Health care structures: the case of Belgium', *Social Science and Medicine* 22: 223–32.

Nys, H. and Quaethoven, P. (1984) 'Health services in Belgium', in M. W. Raffel (ed.), *Comparative Health Systems: Descriptive Analyses of Fourteen National Health Systems*, Pittsburgh: Pennsylvania State University Press.

Pasture, P. (1992) *Kerk, Politiek en Sociale Actie: De Unieke Positie van de Christelijke Arbeidersbeweging in België*, Leuven: Garant.

Schepens, H. (ed.) (1992) *Compendium Gezondheidsstatistiek 1992*, Brussels: BIGE.

Schepers, R. (1979) 'De Orde van Geneesheren: belangenverdediging of deontologie?', *Politica* 29: 130–55.

—— (1993a) 'The Belgian medical profession, the Order of Physicians and the sickness funds (1900–1940)', *Sociology of Health and Illness* 15(3): 375–92.

—— (1993b) 'The Belgian medical profession in a changing society', paper presented at the 'ECPR Session on the State and Health Care', Leiden, 2–8 April.

Therborn, G. (1989) '"Pillarization" and "popular movements". Two variants of welfare state capitalism: the Netherlands and Sweden', in C. G. Castles (ed.), *The Comparative History of Public Policy*, Cambridge: Cambridge University Press.

Vereniging der Belgische Omnipractici (1992) *Riziv-statistieken: Analyse van de VBO*.

Wouters, R., Spinnewyn, H. and Pacolet, J. (1988) *Het Profijt van de Non-profit: De Economische Betekenis van de Gezondheids- en Welzijnszorg*, Brussels: Koning Boudewijnstichting en Hoger Instituut voor de Arbeid.

van der Zee, J., Groenewegen, P. P. and van Haaften, R. (1991) 'Huisartsinkomens in West-Europa', *Nederlands Tijdschrift voor Geneeskunde* 135: 808–13.

11 Midwifery in the Netherlands
More than a semi-profession?

Edwin van Teijlingen and Leonie van der Hulst

Midwifery, nursing and social work are generally considered to be semi-professions (Etzioni 1969). In this chapter we analyse the position of midwifery in the Netherlands and argue that it is more than a semi-profession, that is to say, it has more power and autonomy than midwifery in other industrialized nations *vis-à-vis* the medical profession. We argue that the elevated position of midwives in the Netherlands results from a number of factors, not least the influence of the state on the provision of health care in general and the regulation of health occupations in particular.

What is a semi-profession? While current definitions highlight interrelationships that an occupation has with its clients, competing occupations and the state – that is, adopt a power-based approach – past definitions were derived using a more rigid 'taxonomic approach'. Greenwood (1957), for instance, listed the following qualities required by an occupation if it is to be regarded as a profession:

- systematic theory;
- authority recognized by its clientele;
- broader community sanction;
- code of ethics;
- professional culture sustained by formal professional associations.

Toren (1969: 144) drew on Greenwood's work and thus defined a semi-profession as an occupation in which 'one or more' of the above professional qualities is lacking or is not fully developed. This approach had limitations; for example, midwifery and chiropractic appear to meet the requirements on Greenwood's list, yet they are not recognized as professions. As the list of professional characteristics is extended to exclude non-professions, the approach and resultant definitions become less generally applicable and more specific to a particular time or culture (Richman 1987: 108).

The more recently developed neo-Weberian and Marxist approaches to the professions centre on 'power and control'. Such approaches are more universally applicable than the taxonomic approach. Power and control may be assessed on the basis of some characteristics postulated by the taxonomic approach, and thus the two approaches are not entirely incompatible, but these characteristics are not prescriptive of a profession, only of the power it possesses. Consequently, the definition of a semi-profession is taken as an occupation that is less powerful and has less control than a profession, but is more powerful and has more control than a trade. A semi-profession attempts to exert power over other occupations, clients and the state, but achieves this to a lesser degree than a profession. In short, one can only make comparative statements regarding the professional status of an occupation.

MIDWIFERY IN THE NETHERLANDS

Dutch midwives have been officially recognized as independent medical practitioners since 1865. They can legally practise obstetrics without the supervision of a doctor when pregnancies and deliveries show no indication of medical complications (Smulders and Limburg 1988: 235). In common with most Dutch general practitioners and obstetricians, midwives are self-employed private entrepreneurs rather than salaried employees. Their income consists of the fees they receive from the state health insurance scheme, called the sick funds, and additional fees from private health-insurance companies.

Training takes place at one of the three direct-entry schools of midwifery and lasts three years. It is geared largely towards normal childbirth, but also to selection of pregnant women into different risk categories. Their judgements of risk are guided by a list of 124 medical indications for three well-defined risk levels drawn up by the sick funds (Ziekenfondsraad 1987).

Initially, a pregnant woman is seen by a community midwife, or occasionally by a general practitioner if there is no midwife practising in the region (van Teijlingen and McCaffery 1987). Women in the low-risk category receive antenatal care from the midwife, and delivery will take place at home or, if the woman prefers, during a short-stay hospital delivery. Medium-risk women will at some stage be seen by an obstetrician, but will continue to receive antenatal care from their midwife. These women are strongly advised to deliver in hospital, but they can still be attended by a midwife. If an abnormality presents itself or is likely to do so the pregnancy is defined as high-risk and the woman is referred to an obstetrician for a hospital delivery.

In addition to risk selection, legislation permits midwives to conduct blood tests, to give advice on a suitable diet, to use external manipulation to turn the baby round in the womb and to perform and stitch episiotomies, under local anaesthetics if deemed necessary. Since 1979 the law allows midwives to prescribe a limited number of medicines: such as oxytocine and antirhesus (D) immunoglobine (Klomp 1985: 2127).

During a home birth the midwife will normally be assisted by a maternity home care assistant. In addition, maternity home care assistants assist the midwife by providing care and support for new mothers and their babies for up to eight days after the delivery (van Teijlingen 1990). They provide nursing care to the mother and baby, health education, such as advice on breast-feeding, as well as domestic help in the form of cleaning, shopping or looking after other children in the household. Maternity home care assistants take on the more mundane tasks that elsewhere might be part of the midwife's role.

The preceding profile of the Dutch midwives distinguishes them from most semi-professional midwives in industrialized countries. As independent practitioners, they differ from most of their contemporaries who are in paid employ in a medical hierarchy under a doctor's authority. In Britain, for example, Stacey points out that 'midwives were accepted within the official health-care division of labour but in a position clearly subordinate to medical practitioners' (1988: 78). Nurse-midwives in California are in a similar position, practising in a semi-independent fashion with standardized procedures, but remaining subservient in the medical hierarchy (DeVries 1986: 1148). Dutch midwives are entrepreneurs, while most midwives, in common with nearly all members of the semi-professions, are salaried (Carr-Saunders 1955).

Dutch midwives are trained separately from nurses. Direct-entry midwifery allows the midwives to distinguish themselves from both doctors and nurses and allows them to have their own unique approach to childbirth, based on a psychosocial rather than a medical model. Furthermore, the midwife's sense of professional autonomy is strengthened by the existence of maternity home care assistants, that is to say, they also have some degree of authority over another occupation in their field (van Teijlingen 1990). All these characteristics are indicative of the additional power that Dutch midwives possess in comparison to midwives in other industrialized nations and lend support for the thesis that midwifery in the Netherlands is more than a semi-profession.

The last two centuries have seen Dutch state intervention on a number of occasions to regulate midwifery. We believe it is this intervention, and particularly the supportive form it took, which favoured the midwives as the primary care givers for pregnant women.

STATE INTERVENTION IN MIDWIFERY

Prior to the nineteenth century, regulation of medical occupations in the Netherlands was conducted at the provincial and municipal level, for example the first Dutch municipal regulation of midwifery and of training dates back to 1656 and was drawn up in Delft (Houtzager 1993: 62–4). Following the influence of Napoleon a more centralized state began to emerge and with it national legislation regulating a whole range of occupations. At that time the medical profession remained poorly established, in its infancy in terms of the professionalization process. Thus the modern state developed ahead of the medical profession and sought to bring in legislation which regulated and established the boundaries of professions involved in the provision of medical care, including maternity care.

As early as 1818 the Dutch government introduced a law covering provincial medical examination boards for, among others, midwives. In 1861 professional training was introduced in Amsterdam (van Lieburg and Marland 1989: 306) which institutionalized the position of the midwife (Crébas 1987). Once the state had regulated the midwifery profession each subsequent change in the law would have to take this reality into consideration. In 1865 the Dutch midwife received the status of a practitioner credited with independent clinical judgement, alongside the academically trained doctor. Midwives were the main competitors of general practitioners, since obstetrics had not yet developed as a medical speciality. At the same time major socio-political changes were taking place in Dutch society (Hiddinga 1987: 283). By the turn of the century, local training of maternity home care assistants was being organized in an attempt to reduce the high infant mortality rates that were synonymous with the relatively late industrialization, rapid population increase and poor living conditions. In 1926 the government introduced regulation and training of maternity home care assistants. In so doing the state legitimized an occupation whose role included being an assistant to the midwife and furthermore whose existence was fundamental in enabling birth to remain in the home, traditionally the domain of the midwife. In 1941 the Sick Fund Act was introduced which guaranteed midwives a market share by ruling that general practitioners' fees for providing maternity care are not reimbursed when there is a midwife practising in the area. At the same time, obstetricians' fees are reimbursed only if the physiological process of childbirth turns into a pathological one, or is expected to do so. This financial regulation is of critical importance for Dutch midwives, since it prevents doctors from attending most low-risk births. Since 1941 the range of permitted 'interventions' of midwives has expanded and their skills increased (van der Hulst 1988: 21–2).

DISCUSSION

The supportive intervention for midwifery by the Dutch state is distinctive. In Britain, for example, national legislation was minimal, with the first midwifery act being introduced in England and Wales in 1902, over eighty years after the first Dutch legislation. British legislation also tended to be restrictive, rather than supportive, of midwives' professional development. This indicates the significant input from an already well-organized medical profession in Britain, which sought to restrict the midwives' jurisdiction. It also is consistent with the more general British dislike of government regulations and legislation on issues that can be regulated otherwise (Moran and Wood 1993: 27–8). In the Netherlands the medical profession was regulated when it was still developing, and by the time obstetricians began to establish themselves midwives had already received the status of medical practitioners.

It is not only state intervention which has supported midwives. Another beneficial factor is the existence of maternity home care assistants. We can also analyse their role in the light of the benefits for Dutch midwives. After a home birth the mother and the new-born baby are left in the experienced hands of a maternity home care assistant. 'It relieves midwives of the post-delivery nursing activities', according to community midwives Beatrijs Smulders and Astrid Limburg (1988: 238). Kloosterman also notes that: 'The midwife can devote herself entirely to her obstetric task . . . and is able to take care of 100–200 pregnant women per year' (1978: 86).

A midwife provides postnatal care for those clients for whom she has already provided antenatal and intra-partum care, as well as for women who have delivered in hospital under the care of an obstetrician and have been discharged from hospital. For Dutch midwives postnatal care is less time-consuming than it would be for, for example, British community midwives, since the maternity home care assistant sees the new mother and baby each day during the lying-in period. She monitors the baby's progress, checks the temperature, and so on. The midwife calls in every day after the delivery for four days and then every second day for the next week. If the maternity home care assistant is not satisfied with the condition of the baby and/or the mother she contacts the midwife.

The low status of maternity home care assistants along with their lack of career opportunities puts midwifery automatically higher on the occupational ladder. The very existence of the maternity home care assistant helps to maintain the autonomous position of the Dutch midwife.

PROFESSIONAL COMPETITION

Supportive legislation by itself is not enough for midwives to maintain their independent and autonomous position. For example, in Germany a midwife must be present at every birth by law. However, this has not strengthened the midwifery profession: 'The working situation of midwives is extremely bad. Employed midwives are hopelessly overworked and the units understaffed . . . midwives act as obstetric nurses' (Toussaint 1991: 15). In Britain a similar situation exists. Every pregnant woman has to be allocated a midwife for a home delivery if she so wishes, as mentioned above. But this formal rule does not in practice mean that many pregnant women actually have a home delivery. The system does not facilitate home births, the professionals are very often against it, and public opinion is opposed to it, although the political climate is changing towards supporting midwives, home births and community care, after the publication of several government reports in the early 1990s (House of Commons Health Committee 1992; Expert Maternity Group 1993; Policy Review Group 1993).

In other industrialized countries the most powerful profession of all practitioners in the field of maternity care, the obstetricians, is able to claim jurisdiction over childbirth. Family doctors and midwives ended up in a subordinate position under the control of medical specialists. Obstetricians are at the top of a hierarchy, medically as well as administratively. At this point we would like to introduce Andrew Abbott's model of the 'systems of professions'. Abbott (1988) has argued that inter-professional competition is a fundamental part of professional life. The strongest profession will try to extend its jurisdictional boundaries as widely as possible at the expense of weaker professions.

Economic and ideological motives appeared to be at the foundation of the support for Dutch midwives (van der Hulst 1988). In 1868 there were shortages of midwives as the population began to expand. Doctors were relatively few and they had an interest in keeping midwives as the main birth attendant for the poor.

There were concerns regarding male doctors examining women, a development consistent with the tightening of moral values towards the end of the century. A lack of female obstetricians and doctors made the midwife the obvious choice. Consequently, a somewhat unusual relationship prevailed between some obstetricians, midwifery and the state. Rather than lobbying against midwives in the late nineteenth century, some prominent obstetricians 'advocated the cause of the Dutch midwife and, as a result, the Government extended the education of midwives from two to three years, and incorporated prenatal care' (Smulders and Limburg 1988: 238). Professor Kloosterman fulfilled a similar role in the 1960s, 1970s and 1980s, and his successor at the University of Amsterdam, Professor Treffers, continues the tradition of promoting midwifery and the availability of home birth as an option. Within the national association, the obstetricians remain divided on the issue. Until recently Dutch obstetricians have had a fairly protective attitude towards midwives (Lems 1986: 27).

MEDICAL DOMINANCE

Turner argues that: 'In the health field, medical dominance is a necessary feature of the professional power and superiority of the medical practitioner in relation to other occupations' (1987: 141). He identifies three modes of dominance over allied occupations, namely subordination, limitation and exclusion. The third of these forms of medical dominance involves denying potential competitors access to the benefits of registration and legitimate status: an example would be that lay midwifery is illegal in some states of the United States (DeVries 1986). Limitation implies a containment to just one part of the body (dentists) or of the life-cycle (Dutch midwives), or to a specific therapeutic method (pharmacists). Finally, subordination describes a situation in which an occupation is controlled and regulated by a medical profession, for instance midwifery in Britain and nursing in general.

In this chapter we are interested in the historical development of the present relationships between the care providers in the maternity services. Abbott's model of the 'systems of professions' offers insight into this process. He has argued that the evolution of professions in fact result from their interrelations. 'These interrelations are in turn determined by the way these groups control their knowledge and skills' (Abbott 1988: 8). This link between a profession and its work, a link which Abbott analyses in terms of jurisdiction, is a central phenomenon of professional life. Jurisdiction is a more-or-less exclusive claim, every move in one profession's jurisdiction affects those of others in the system. Dominance is an important system property; it may be 'structural-control of organizations and institutions. It may be cultural-control of dominant ideas. It may be both' (Abbott 1988: 109).

In most countries obstetricians dominate both the structure and the culture of the provision of maternity care, while the Dutch obstetricians can be seen as having considerable structural dominance, but not cultural dominance. The generally accepted idea in the Netherlands that home birth is safe unless contraindications exist reflects a psycho-social model of childbirth, not a medical model. Crébas (1987) notes that Dutch midwives have their own jurisdiction: over normal childbirth. They emphasize their expertise in the psycho-social approach domain, an expertise which is geared to a holistic approach to antenatal and perinatal care, whereas the obstetrical profession is dominated by a medicalized model of childbirth.

The different government approaches to professions have contributed to the existing differences in available maternity care. The state overshadows professional life in continental countries. As Abbott says: 'The different relationship between authority and obligation is one of the profound differences between continental and Anglo-American professions' (1988: 60). The continental professions are regulated and limited by the state, whilst in America and Britain general social obligations are merely based on codes of professional ethics. However, this continental limitation by the state can very well act as a protection for the regulated profession against competitors. Thus when the state grants one particular profession a licensed right to do certain work, others are excluded. Dutch midwives are a perfect example of this thesis. They are limited to attending 'low-risk' pregnant women and they are not allowed to do instrumental deliveries. This considerably restricts their jurisdiction in the total provision of maternity care. However, at the same time it excludes other professions from invading their jurisdiction: general practitioners are not reimbursed for providing maternity care in areas where a midwife is practising, and obstetricians are not reimbursed for attending 'low-risk' deliveries. The Dutch maintained their particular organization of maternity care, partly for ideological motives, and partly for financial motives. As Torres and Reich note, the Dutch government 'has sought to regulate essential but specific aspects of the health system, particularly those related to rising costs' (1989: 409).

It should therefore not be surprising that the Dutch government promotes home births attended by midwives or family doctors as its policy is to move care out of the hospital into the home. It still recognizes that home birth is a normal and accepted phenomenon which depends upon the existence of a system of maternity home care assistance, the well-trained independent midwife and, moreover, that the Dutch system is cheaper than that of its neighbours (Simons 1991: 20). In addition, all the major political parties, from the left to the right, agree that the midwife is the obvious person to provide maternity care, and that deliveries should preferably take place at home (Tweede Kamer der Staten-Generaal 1990).

CONCLUSION

In a sense one could argue that Abbott's theory, with regard to the continental professions, centres on explaining the different systems of professions in France (and by implication, the Netherlands) in terms of a different culture and a different state structure. The professions as such are not different in their development and their constant competition to maintain and expand their jurisdiction: the difference lies in the state as an intervening variable.

In the Netherlands the different professional groups are more equally balanced; the balance of power does not lie in the hands of one particular group of practitioners. Direct and indirect state intervention in the provision of maternity care has been extremely supportive of the independent midwives. Abbott's analysis helps us to understand the impact of state actions on the outcome of competition between professional groups in a 'system of professions'.

Crébas has argued that in the Netherlands 'midwifery is a medical profession in a legal sense and a semi-profession in a sociological sense' (1986: 48). We would argue that Dutch midwifery is more than a semi-profession in a sociological sense. Government support for the organization of maternity care with its large proportion of home births and short-stay hospital deliveries attended by midwives and family doctors, together with the aforementioned factors, seems to put midwives in the Netherlands in a different analytical category compared to the traditional semi-professions. The state has somehow limited the power of the profession of obstetrics in the Netherlands and thus as a power broker has allowed midwives more power and autonomy than their counterparts in other industrialized countries.

ACKNOWLEDGEMENTS

The authors would like to thank Annette Ross for proof-reading this chapter and for her constructive criticism on earlier drafts.

REFERENCES

Abbott, A. (1988) *The System of Professions: An Essay on the Division of Expert Labor*, Chicago: University of Chicago Press.

Carr-Saunders, A. M. (1955) 'Metropolitan conditions and traditional professional relationships', in R. M. Fisher (ed.), *The Metropolis in Modern Life*, New York: Doubleday.

Crébas, A. (1986) *De Positie van de Zelfstandig Gevestigde Verloskundige in Nederland: Een Verkennende Literatuurstudie*, Amsterdam: Werkgroep Verloskunde '78.

—— (1987) 'De natuurlijke geboorte in Nederland en de beroepsidentiteit van de zelfstandig gevestigde verloskundige', *Tijdschrift voor Verloskundigen* 12: 121–4.

DeVries, R. G. (1986) 'The contest for control: regulating new and expanding health occupations', *American Journal of Public Health* 76(9): 1147–50.

Etzioni, A. (ed.) (1969) *The Semi-Professions and their Organization*, New York: Free Press.

Expert Maternity Group (1993) *Changing Childbirth*, Part 1, London: HMSO.

Freidson, E. (1970) *Profession of Medicine: A Study of the Sociology of Applied Knowledge*, New York: Dodd, Mead & Co.

Greenwood, E. (1957) 'Attributes of a profession', *Social Work* 2: 45–55.

Hiddinga, A. (1987) 'Obstetrical research in the Netherlands in the 19th century', *Medical History* 31: 281–305.

House of Commons Health Committee (1992) *Second Report: Maternity Services* 1, London: HMSO.

Houtzager, H. L. (1993) *Wat er in de Kraam te Pas Komt: Opstellen Over de Geschiedenis van de Verloskunde in Nederland*, Rotterdam: Erasmus Publishing.

van der Hulst, L. (1988) 'Vroedvrouw een veranderende status', dissertation, University of Amsterdam.

—— (1989) 'Vroedvrouw en "Dekker"', *Medisch Contact* 45: 1489–92.

Klomp, J. (1985) 'De wettelijke bevoegdheden van de verloskundige', *Nederlands Tijdschrift voor Geneeskunde* 129: 2125–8.

Kloosterman, G. J. (1978) 'The Dutch system of home births', in S. Kitzinger and J. Davis (eds), *The Place of Birth*, Oxford: Oxford University Press.

Lems, A. A. (1986) 'Verloskundigen willen zelfstandigheid versterken', *Inzet* 9: 26–7.

van Lieburg, M. J. and Marland, H. (1989) 'Midwife regulation, education, and practice in the Netherlands during the nineteenth century', *Medical History* 33: 296–317.

Lorentzon, M. (1990) 'Professional status and managerial tasks: feminine service ideology in British nursing and social work', in P. Abbott and C. Wallace (eds), *The Sociology of the Caring Professions*, London: Falmer Press.

Moran, M. and Wood, B. (1993) *States, Regulation and the Medical Profession*, Buckingham: Open University Press.

Policy Review Group (1993) *Provision of Maternity Services in Scotland: A Policy Review*, Edinburgh: HMSO.

Richman, J. (1987) *Medicine and Health*, London: Longman.

Simons, H. (1991) 'De verloskundige: spil of speelbal?', in L. van der Hulst (ed.), *De Vroedvrouw, de Spil van de Verloskunde*, Bilthoven: Catherina Schrader Stichting.

Smulders, B. and Limburg, A. (1988) 'Obstetrics and midwifery in the Netherlands', in S. Kitzinger (ed.), *The Midwife Challenge*, London: Pandora.

Stacey, M. (1988) *The Sociology of Health and Healing: A Textbook*, London: Unwin Hyman.

van Teijlingen, E. R. (1990) 'The profession of maternity home care assistant and its significance for the Dutch midwifery profession', *International Journal of Nursing Studies* 27: 355–66.

van Teijlingen, E. R. and McCaffery, P. (1987) 'The profession of midwife in the Netherlands', *Midwifery* 3: 178–86.

Toren, N. (1969) 'Semi-professionalism and social work: a theoretical perspective', in A. Etzioni (ed.), *The Semi-Professions and their Organization*, New York: Free Press.

Torres, A. and Reich, M. R. (1989) 'The shift from home to institutional childbirth: a comparative study of the United Kingdom and the Netherlands', *International Journal of Health Services* 3: 405–14.

Toussaint, J. (1991) 'Midwifery in Germany Part 1', *MIDIRS Midwifery Digest* 1: 15–16.

Turner, B. S. (1987) *Medical Power and Social Knowledge*, London: Sage.

Tweede Kamer der Staten-Generaal (1990) *Vaststelling van de Begroting van de Uitgaven en de Ontvangsten van Hoofdstuk XVI (Ministerie van Welzijn, Volksgezondheid en Cultuur) voor het Jaar 1990: Tweede Kamer 1989–1990*, 21 300 XVI No. 42, The Hague: SDU Uitgeverij.

Ziekenfondsraad (1987) *De Verloskundige Indicatielijst*, Amstelveen: Ziekenfondsraad.

12 State traditions and medical professionalization in Scandinavia

Vibeke Erichsen

The 1980s saw a proliferation of scholarly work specifying national particularities in the historical development of professions. Moves have been taken towards developing theoretical analyses that can accommodate both historical and comparative evidence (Burrage *et al.* 1990). Typically contrasted in the literature are the practitioner-led processes found in countries such as England and the United States versus the more state-led patterns of France and other continental societies.

As yet little research has been undertaken in order to locate the Scandinavian countries in relation to the two proposed models of professionalization. An interesting departure has been made by Torstendahl (1985). On the one hand, the fact that the state in Scandinavia typically is active and fairly strong more than suggests that professionalization comes close to a state-led model. On the other hand, if we accept the notion of the Scandinavian welfare state as a particular state structure characterized by large public bureaucracies consisting of a large proportion of professionals making a significant imprint on policies (Esping-Andersen 1990; Kolberg 1991; Erichsen 1993; Nordby 1993), there are indications of patterns of professionalization that somewhat differ from the state-led models of the Continent. Whether Scandinavia has experienced a particular type of state-led development or somehow has been shaped between a state-led and practitioner-led model is premature to assess.

This chapter is a preliminary exercise in particularizing Scandinavian developments, with its point of departure in the medical profession. The very notion of a Scandinavian model is of course blind to significant differences between Sweden, Norway and Denmark. More important in this context however, are, the structures and experiences shared by the Scandinavian countries. Employing empirical evidence from Sweden and Norway, the chapter will explore the ways in which articulation between the state and the medical profession has been shaped historically. It can offer only a preliminary scrutiny of various forms, and processes of articulation, as efforts to locate the Scandinavian experience(s) in the wider international picture have just started.

PROFESSIONS AND STATE STRUCTURES

The mainstream literature on the professions typically misconceives the relationship between professions and the state. The state and the professions tend to be seen as antithetical phenomena. Implicit is the notion of bureaucracy versus profession, and state intervention versus professional autonomy. State bureaucracies and other bureaucratic structures are seen as threats to professional autonomy. Terry Johnson argued to the contrary when he claimed that a close relationship of a profession to the state apparatus 'may constitute the very conditions within which occupational autonomy is possible' (1982: 189). Over a decade later, with the state intervention/professional autonomy controversy still unresolved in the sociology of professions, he develops further in this volume the argument that state formation in the modern world includes the professions, thus eliminating the profession/state duality.

Perhaps surprisingly the state/profession duality survived well during the 1980s despite the departure from universalizing, 'one route' theories of professionalization as formulated by scholars of the functionalist school. Notions of professionalization as practitioner-led and state-led potentially imply a recognition that processes of professionalization follow fundamentally different routes that are bound in time and place. By implication professional autonomy and state intervention cannot be seen as antithetical concepts. Very different processes of professionalization – including those that are 'state-near' – might give rise to powerful, though differently constituted, professions. Bureaucratization, state-making and professionalization should thus be seen as interrelated, and indeed interdependent, processes.

As yet these new departures have not had much of an impact on the understanding of Scandinavian circumstances. For instance, scholars have argued that the rise of the Swedish welfare state has dramatically undermined the power of the medical profession. An illuminating example is Arnold Heidenheimer, who argues that 'it has been during the past quarter century that many aspects of professional autonomy have become more circumscribed in Sweden than elsewhere in the West' (1980: 119). The opposite conclusion has been reached by the Swedish scholar Karin Johannisson, when she writes that the Swedish public health project was

> guided by strong governmental involvement, embracing the medical profession itself. It is generally acknowledged that the status of the medical profession is reduced in proportion to the degree of state intervention. In Sweden, this is not the case – though 85 per cent of the physicians are publicly employed – mainly because of an historical tradition, in which the central authority acknowledged its need for physicians to supervise the health of a nation characterized by low population density and modest urbanization levels by giving these doctors social security, influence and prestige in turn.
>
> (1991: 23)

There is undoubtedly a need for theoretical and empirical clarification.

It is my impression that although scholars might recognize professionalization as a multi-route project, the tendency remains for questions still to be posed within a theoretical framework which sees professions as pressure groups. This implies that questions are mainly asked about the autonomy of professions in relation to the state, and how they exert power to influence the regulation of professional activities. Health policies would be interpreted as state interventions in the market and professional associations would be the primary object of analysis. In short, professions are seen as interest groups external to the state apparatus itself. Very different questions spring from what we might call a statist perspective. At the core would be questions relating to professional authority in policy-making. These focus on ways in which professions identify problems and solutions associated with public policies, how they contribute to ideological hegemonies, and to the definition of relevant knowledge and values (Erichsen 1993: 395). The medical profession, or more notably segments of it, would by their nearness to public bureaucracies be expected to exert influence on health policies by providing information and expert analysis. Of no less importance, respect for medical knowledge might be used to influence ways of thinking and thus the priorities of public policies. To a much larger extent than is seen in the scholarly literature, professions should be analysed as an integrated part of the state itself.

While the concepts of autonomy and authority are often used interchangeably in the literature on professions, the above discussion suggests that a statist mode of analysis will be concerned more with authority than autonomy and, vice versa, that a pressure group perspective tends to emphasize profession-led patterns and autonomy more than authority. The term professional autonomy typically refers to the ability of doctors to make autonomous decisions concerning the content and conditions of the process involved in medical work (Freidson 1970b: 368). As proposed by Freidson and others, there are thus political, economic and clinical aspects of professional autonomy (Freidson 1970a; Elston 1991: 61). Legal-rational authority relates in a Weberian sense to a bureaucratic structure. The present analysis will follow Talcott Parsons (1964: 59) in emphasizing that legal-rational authority should be seen as embracing authority arising from both 'legal competence' and 'technical competence'. In the analysis of professions and the state professional authority should be seen as composed of both aspects. Professional authority is thus viewed as socially sanctioned expertise employed in the hands of the state.

The present analysis of Scandinavian experiences will draw on statist analysis and focus on aspects of professional authority, seeing these as particularly significant for our understanding of medical professionalization in Scandinavia. For this purpose it might be fruitful to distinguish between three spheres of medical authority in state–profession relationships:

1 The relationship of doctors to other key actors within the political-administrative apparatus of the state, at central and local levels of government. Coalitions, control and compromise in these relationships are essential to such an analysis.

2   The internal dynamics of the medical profession which are most significantly expressed in the relationship between hospital-based medicine and general practice. Health care systems vary greatly as to the degree of hospital-centredness across both time and space. The term 'hospital-centredness' refers to the proportion of health care resources going into the hospitals. The more hospital-centred a health care system is, the more predominant ideas and norms associated with high-technology medicine are expected to be (Davies 1979).

3   The external dynamics of medicine which involve the division of labour, and most typically the gendered division of labour in medicine. It should not be taken for granted that the change over time from extensive medical dominance in a rather simple division of labour to a less dominant, or even negotiated, role in a much more complex division of labour necessarily implies a decline in medical authority.

The historical analysis that we shall now turn to examines the ways in which these three spheres of medical authority have been expressed in state–profession relationships in Scandinavia over time. Following the analytical perspective introduced above, medical professionalization will be analysed as part of state formation. A few words should be said about the concept of the state that underpins such an enterprise. In a Weberian perspective the state is seen as consisting of sets of interdependent institutions making up a (semi-)autonomous state. Particularly consistent with the concept of professionalization that has been forwarded above is a state concept which takes into consideration the ways in which interest representation and state autonomy fit together. Such a concept is embedded in the work of Bo Straath and Rolf Torstendahl (1992) when they propose that the state should be seen as a network structure. The structure is logically separate from individual action, albeit treated as coming about only via the interrelationship of individual actions. Accordingly, the key focus in an analysis of state formation would be transitional periods in which social interests are pulled into the state or changes in interrelationships in other respects occur. Singled out for investigation are two particularly significant historical periods. The reader should be warned that this constitutes a very simple analytical framework which does not amount to a theory of state formation/professionalization, nor does it impose a strict chronological sequence. Developed in the following sections are some broad conceptions of, first, the historical development of state–profession relationships in the bourgeois-bureaucratic state until the opening of the twentieth century, and, second, medical professionalization in the social democratic era. The concluding section discusses the prospects for medicine in the restructured Scandinavian welfare state. What is offered here is thus a rough sketch of some broad historical trends that need to be painted in order to picture state–profession relationships in Scandinavia. Needless to say, things are far from as tidy as the sketch suggests.

MEDICAL AUTHORITY IN THE BOURGEOIS-BUREAUCRATIC STATE

The close interweaving of state-making and the development of the medical profession is perhaps most interestingly demonstrated by students of the early Swedish medical administration. During this period Sweden emerged as a monarchical bureaucratic regime, to be rapidly transformed into an industrialist-capitalist parliamentary democracy – the bourgeois-bureaucratic state – a process which was completed in the early twentieth century (Weir and Skocpol 1985; Therborn 1989).

Established in the seventeenth century, the *Collegium Medicum* (College of Medicine) was in Sweden a corporate organ granting to physicians self-regulation and the right to exercise certain powers in relation to other health occupations. The state also put in the hands of the College some control of the health services. The role of the College gradually expanded from being advisory, then regulatory, to finally being involved in policy-making (Kearns *et al.* 1989: 32). Increasingly it became part of the domain of the state. The first step in the transformation took place in 1813, when the College became part of the collegiate structure of central government (*Sundhetscollegium*). A second step was taken in 1878 when the National Board of Health (*Medicinalstyrelsen*) was created, implying the replacement of the previous collegiate order with the hierarchical model of bureaucracy (Gustafsson 1987; Garpenby 1989; Rogers and Nelson 1989).

A clear continuity thus existed between the mercantilistic state and the health administration of the bourgeois-bureaucratic state of nineteenth-century Sweden. The incorporation into the bureaucratic state of a corporate professional body contrasts strikingly with the British case. The corporate structure of the British medical profession has survived fairly well in the Royal Colleges. It is a corporate structure external to the state, not within the state, as in Sweden. The Norwegian case resembles that of Sweden, although with certain modifications, as indicated by the controversies over collegiate medical administration in the 1840s, and the fact that a (semi-)autonomous unit within central government was not established until 1892 (Benum 1979; Maurseth 1979; Berg 1991).

That the integration of the medical profession into the state was strong compared to Britain seems clear from this account. In order to distinguish the Scandinavian type of integration from that of continental Europe, we may draw on classifications developed by Rolf Torstendahl (1991: 36). He describes nineteenth-century Sweden as a highly centralized state with a high degree of bureaucratization. This contrasts with Germany (low centralization, high bureaucratization) and France (high centralization, low bureaucratization). If we add to this picture that Sweden and Norway have in common with Germany a juridical bureaucratic tradition, it should come as no surprise that the process of incorporation involved at the central level of government fuelled conflicts between doctors and lawyers. Thus the medical profession during the early stages of its professionalization became part of a highly centralized and bureaucratized state apparatus. Simultaneously institutionalized during this process were tensions in medical administration between lawyers and medical doctors.

Locally the incorporation of doctors found expression in the establishment of health boards, from 1860 in Norway and 1874 in Sweden. They defined a key role for doctors in both countries in public health. In Norway the district doctor was designated by law to act as chairman of the local health board, and also in Sweden a doctor in state employment was typically found as chairman (Seip 1984; Larsen and Hodne 1988).

The local health service could be described as an extension of the central government health administration (Berg 1991). Certain variations existed between urban areas, where doctors generally could sustain some private practice, at least in combination with public employment, and rural areas, where in Sweden in 1773 doctors were made state employees (Bergstrand 1963). A comparative analysis of nineteenth-century urban public health policies in Germany, England and Sweden concluded that:

> The reliance of the Swedish medical sector on state patronage is staggering. In many ways the Swedish case was professional fulfilment. A clear commitment by the state to stand by the self-regulation of the profession was supplemented by the provision of appropriate posts.
>
> (Kearns *et al.* 1989: 24–5)

In Norway the situation was similar to Sweden, as noted by Ole Berg: 'Doctors could only move out [from cities] with the aid of the state, as public doctors, and increasingly, the medical profession succeeded in having the state establish public physician posts in rural areas' (1980: 35).

From very different institutional frameworks, hospital doctors emerged in both Britain and France as the élite within the medical profession (Jamous and Peloille 1970; Honigsbaum 1979). Certain differences between Sweden and Norway ought to be taken into consideration when trying to establish the role of the hospital in medical professionalization in Scandinavia. At the end of the nineteenth century Sweden had a more hospital-centred health system than Norway; one in five and one in ten doctors respectively was in hospital employment (Berg 1980). Rooted in Sweden's history as a military power, the difference in terms of hospital-centredness was probably reinforced from the late eighteenth century, when hospital care was administratively separated from poor relief and placed under central control. Similar steps were not taken in Norway, where hospitals 'were often intimately linked to the work for the poor, or they were special-disease institutions – like the leproseries. There was no central co-ordination and control of these institutions' (Berg 1980: 40).

Closer links between the state and hospitals were thus established in Sweden than in Norway. That the Swedish state relied extensively on policies directed at individual cases of sickness, directed towards hospitals (Kearns *et al.* 1989: 34), is an indication that the integration of medicine into the bourgeois-bureaucratic state strengthened medical authority.

That the hospital system hardly contributed to the production of a professional

Table 12.1 Population per doctor and midwife, 1850 and 1900

| | Doctor | | Midwife | |
	1850	1900	1850	1900
Norway	4,800[1]	2,519	3,306[1]	1,959
Sweden	7,522	3,845	2,531	1,846
England	1,176	1,433	8,857	10,604

1   1860.

Sources: Statistiska Centralbyrån (1969), Statistisk Sentralbyrå (1978), Kearns *et al.* (1989).

élite in Norway, nor in Sweden, might be due to the fact that the hospitals were largely served by the public district doctors, and to their separation from medical educational institutions. That the state universities were the only training institutions for doctors, and that faculty doctors acted as advisers to the government and sometimes also as chairmen of local health boards were factors contributing to the constitution of faculty doctors as the medical élite in Sweden and Norway (Berg 1986; Nelson 1992).

We shall now examine the third sphere of medical authority, as identified in the previous section. An interesting starting point for discussion are the differences between England, Sweden and Norway in terms of the division of labour between doctors and midwives, as shown in Table 12.1. The English figures indicate that between 1850 and 1900 the rapidly expanding category of general medical practitioners took over from midwives the larger part of work related to childbirth. This marked the start of the 'medicalization of childbirth' (Lewis 1980). How should the contrasting patterns found in Sweden and Norway be interpreted in this context? Whilst in England during the latter half of the nineteenth century the part played by midwives in childbirth was dramatically reduced, an opposite move apparently took place in Sweden and Norway. On one hand, the increasing density of midwives might indicate that doctors were losing control of the medical division of labour. On the other, both doctors and midwives worked as state employees, with midwives formally subordinated to doctors. Doctors were also in complete control of the training of midwives (Kjaerheim 1980; Blom 1987). It might be argued, therefore, that their close links with the state sustained the control of doctors over the medical division of labour. It should, however, be noted that the fact that doctors were few, especially in Sweden, restricted their ability to keep a close eye on the day-to-day work of midwives. If not formally, in practice midwives were thus likely to enjoy some autonomy in their work.

MEDICINE AND THE SOCIAL DEMOCRATIC WELFARE STATE

Sweeping across Western industrial democracies in the 1930s, the Great Depression gave room in many countries for the development of very close ties between scientific communities and the state. In Sweden and Norway these developments coincided with the rise of social democracy. It has been argued that in Scandinavia the centralized and bureaucratically anchored pattern of policy-making provided ready access for interest groups and experts on strategic decisions (Weir and Skocpol 1985). Various policy fields, from macroeconomic management to health care, experienced the marriage of scientific ideas to social democratic policy-making.

A most notable regime of expert rule developed in Norwegian health care under Karl Evang. A key figure in the Socialist Doctors' Association and a social democrat, and in 1938 appointed Director of the Board of Health, he was for decades the top bureaucrat in health care (Nordby 1989). In the Evang era the prolonged and intense struggles between lawyers and doctors in health administration came to a head and the hegemony of lawyers was brought to an end (Nordby 1987). The success of Evang in implementing his health administrative programme rested to a large extent upon his strong bureaucratic role and also the careful steps he took not to antagonize the various branches of the medical profession. An important factor contributing to the latter relates to the occupation of Norway by Germany during the war. Various groups of doctors and politicians across political party lines were brought together in the course of the war, both in the resistance movement in Norway, and in Norwegian settlements abroad. The Evang era saw medical doctors at the apex of a system of specialized knowledge that was to a large extent integrated with the bureaucratic apparatus of the state.

Whilst the style of Norwegian health policy in the early postwar period might be described as one of establishing consensus through cooperation and compromise, the Swedish style was apparently characterized by a certain degree of confrontation between the government and the medical association. In that country consensus was established through coercion (Garpenby 1989: 208).

The close web of relationships that were formed in Norway between doctors and the social democratic state in the early post-Second World War period did not come about in Sweden until the late 1960s. Two interrelated processes took place from about 1960. First, the health sector, and most notably the hospitals, experienced an enormous growth rate, turning Sweden into not only the 'most rapidly growing Western system' (Heidenheimer 1980: 119), but also the most hospital-centred of all OECD countries, followed closely by Norway at least until the late 1970s. Around the mid-1980s some 73 per cent of the total health care expenditure went into hospitals in Sweden, compared to almost 70 per cent in Norway, the OECD mean being 54 per cent (OECD 1987; see also Tengvald 1988).

The second process involved a restructuring of the medical élite. It is probably a fair contention that the creation of a hospital-based élite within the medical profession coincided in Sweden and Norway with the rise of the social democratic state. Whilst in the bourgeois-bureaucratic state university professors typically constituted the élite, by virtue of being advisers and policy-makers in the state bureaucracy, and in some instances also locally on the health boards, the increasing significance of hospital-based medicine gradually caused a change. The hospital-based specialists (consultants) emerged as the new élite. In Sweden their power also rested on the system of out-patient departments attached to hospitals, providing consultants with a basis for private activities. In the 1950s, the number of visits to the out-patient departments continued to increase, as did the incomes of the consultants. The 1959 Hospital Act, and later the controversial Seven Crowns Reform introduced in 1970, put an end to the right of consultants to collect fees from patients. Hospital doctors were thus made whole-time salaried staff. In the medical profession those favouring these changes were mainly to be found among younger doctors (Garpenby 1989: 163). Their growing significance is expressed well in the relative distribution of representatives from the two groups on the Swedish Medical Association Executive Committee. The ratio, which in 1950 was 7:1 in favour of the consultants, had in 1975 changed to 6:5 in favour of junior doctors (Heidenheimer 1980: 126).

It might be argued, therefore, that what took place in the years leading up to 1970 was not primarily a circumscription of professional autonomy, as argued by amongst others Heidenheimer (1980), but changes in the balance of power within the hospital-based medical élite. It seems fair to say that an implicit coalition emerged between junior hospital-based doctors and the social democratic state. Thus medicine became incorporated into the social democratic state.

In Sweden, to a larger extent than in Norway, it has proved virtually impossible to modify the extreme hospital-centredness of the health system. Already in a 1958 government report concern was expressed over hospital bias, 'however, the wish for a better balance between hospital service . . . was not put into effect' (Garpenby 1989: 87). Ten years later another government report emphasized the need for a transfer of resources from hospitals in the acute sector towards chronic and non-institutional care. In 1990 no changes had taken place (Järnebeck and Laxhed 1990/1: 97,98). A recent review of the Swedish health sector suggests that the counties are under pressure from the medical profession to preserve the extreme hospital-centred system (Järnebeck and Laxhed 1990/1: 123). Norway, experiencing a rapid growth of hospitals following the 1969 Hospital Act which transferred hospitals to the counties (Hansen 1979; Martinsen 1989), has succeeded in reducing the hospital bias somewhat from the late 1970s, and most notably after the establishment in 1984 of local authority-based primary care. Table 12.2 indicates the situation by the mid-1980s.

Although it is beyond this analysis to examine in any detail the factors contributing to the hospital-centredness of Scandinavian health care systems, the

Table 12.2 Institutional loci of medical work, 1985 (%)

	Sweden	Norway
Hospitals	65	50
General practice	29	39
Other	6	11

Sources: Adapted from Riska (1988: 140) and Statistiska Centralbyrån (1991/2: 149).

combined effect of strong planning and policy-making medical administrative units at the central level of government, the emergence of hospital doctors as the new medical élite and the decentralized hospital structure should be noted. As a result there has been a significant penetration of dominant ideas and knowledge associated with high-technology medicine. While the relationship of medicine to nursing in the bourgeois-bureaucratic state was characterized by subordination as defined via the centralized state, the social democratic era saw changes in this relationship in two respects. First, subordination increasingly had its roots in the hospital-centredness of the health care system, and, second, the professionalization of nursing took place within a biomedical framework.

MEDICINE IN TRADITION: THE PAST IN THE PRESENT

The argument has been put forward that there was a continuity between the role of experts during the rise in the 1930s of social democracy and its postwar heyday. Moreover, it has been argued that such continuity can be traced back to historical developments in medical administration, laid down from the seventeenth century onwards (Qvarsell 1992). We would expect, then, that the historical patterns in medical professionalization as they have been identified and discussed in this chapter constitute a legacy relevant to our understanding of contemporary circumstances.

Quests for cost-containment, consumer choice and user participation in health care have in recent years led to the establishment in some countries of 'provider markets'. Similar developments can be seen in the Scandinavian countries. Sweden is embarking on large-scale market reforms. In Norway experiments have started in one county and in central government a proposal for financial and organizational reform is presently under preparation, to be presented to Parliament in 1994.

An intriguing question is whether the new directions that health policy might take will lead to fundamental changes in the constitution of the medical profession. Will the medical profession in Scandinavia change from being constituted as a state-near profession drawing authority and autonomy from its close relationship with the state, to becoming more of a market-shaped profession? In other words, will there be a transition from a state-led to a provider-led, or even market-led medical professionalization? As yet it is premature to assess the impact of reform. However, it seems fair to suggest that issues and tensions that emerged during the 1980s will have an imprint on further developments.

In Norway a reorganization of health care administration in central government apparently led to a reconstruction of expertise in health care. Old tensions between medical and judicial expertise have reappeared, and a reversal of power relations seems to be the outcome. Increasingly economists and political scientists are also replacing doctors as health policy experts. This trend is noticeable in the preparations for reform already mentioned, where doctors are substituted by social scientists. In hospitals the hegemony of doctors has been challenged by the rise of 'new' management. There are also indications that changes are underway in the relationship between nurses and doctors in hospitals, as it has now become possible for nurses to become heads of hospital departments. This is a development trend particular to Norway. In Sweden legislation has recently reinforced the subordination of nurses to doctors in hospital management (Sommervold 1993). While policies of reform might lead to a restructuring of the medical profession, as suggested above, the opposite effect should not be ruled out. In other words, the particular interweaving of the state and the medical profession in Scandinavia might well shape the process of health care reform and thus modify market reforms and reinforce state regulation of the health services.

ACKNOWLEDGEMENTS

This chapter stems from a research project on the social organization of health care, funded by the Norwegian Research Council. An earlier version of this chapter was read at a conference on 'Social Ingeniörkunst i Teori och Praktik' at Linköping in June 1992. The author is indebted to Boel Berner for helpful comments on the earlier draft.

REFERENCES

Benum, E. (1979) *Sentraladministrasjonens Historie, Bind 2, 1845–1884*, Oslo: Universitetsforlaget.

Berg, O. (1973) *Medisinen som Samfunnsinstitusjon*, Department of Political Science, University of Oslo.

—— (1980) 'The modernisation of medical care in Sweden and Norway', in A. J. Heidenheimer and N. Elvander (eds), *The Shaping of the Swedish Health System*, London: Sage.

—— (1986) 'Verdier og interesser – den norske lægeforenings fremvekst og utvikling', in O. Larsen, P. Berg and F. Hodne (eds), *Legene og Samfunnet*, Oslo.

—— (1991) 'Mediakrati, hierarki og marked', in D. Album and G. Midre (eds), *Mellom Idealer og Realiteter: Studier i Medisinsk Sosiologi*, Oslo: Ad Notam.

Bergstrand, H. (1963) 'Läkarekaaren och provinsial-läkareväsendet', in W. Kock (ed.), (1963) *Medicinalväsenet i Sverige 1813–1963*, Stockholm: Nordiska Bokhandelns Förlag.

Blom, I. (1987) 'Sykehusfödsler paa 1800-tallet', *Historisk tidsskrift* 3: 324–44.

Burrage, M., Jarausch, K. and Siegrist, H. (1990) 'An actor-based framework for the study of the professions', in M. Burrage and R. Torstendahl (eds), *Professions in Theory and History. Rethinking the Study of the Professions*, London: Sage.

Davies, C. (1979) 'Hospital-centred health care: policies and politics in the NHS', in P. Atkinson, R. Dingwall and A. Murcott (eds), *Prospects for the National Health*, London: Croom Helm.

Elston, M. A. (1991) 'The politics of professional power: medicine in a changing health service', in J. Gabe, M. Calnan and M. Bury (eds), *The Sociology of the Health Service*, London: Routledge.

Erichsen, V. (1993) 'States and health care: Scandinavian welfare state research', in M. Moran (ed.), *European Journal of Political Research: Annual Review*, Antwerp: Kluwer.

Esping-Andersen, G. (1990) *The Three Worlds of Welfare Capitalism*, Princeton, New Jersey: Princeton University Press.

Freidson, E. (1970a) *Profession of Medicine: A Study in the Sociology of Applied Knowledge*, New York: Dodd, Mead & Co.

—— (1970b) *Professional Dominance: The Social Structure of Medical Care*, New York: Atherton.

Garpenby, P. (1989) *The State and the Medical Profession: A Cross-National Comparison of the Health Policy Arena in the United Kingdom and Sweden 1945–1985*, Linköping: Linköping Studies in Arts and Science.

Gustafsson, R. A. (1987) *Traditionernas ok: Den Svenska Hälso- och Sjukvårdens Organisering i Historie-sociologisk Perspektiv*, Stockholm: Esselte Studium.

Hansen, F. H. (1979) 'Helsesektoren i velferdsstaten: kjempevekst og fordelingskrise', *Tidsskrift for Samfunnsforskning* 20: 219–40.

Heidenheimer, A. J. (1980) 'Conflict and compromises between professional and bureaucratic health interests', in A. J. Heidenheimer and N. Elvander (eds), *The Shaping of the Swedish Health System*, London: Sage.

Honigsbaum, F. (1979) *The Division in British Medicine*, London: Kogan Page.

Jamous, H. and Peloille, B. (1970) 'Professions or self-perpetuating systems? Changes in the French university-hospital system', in J. A. Jackson (ed.), *Professions and Professionalization*, Cambridge: Cambridge University Press.

Järnebeck, G. and Laxhed, I. (1990/1) *Den Svenska Hälso- och Sjukvården*, Stockholm: Riksdagens Revisorer, Rapport No. 4.

Johannisson, K. (1991) 'The people's health: public health in Sweden', paper presented at conference on the 'History of Public Health and Prevention', Lidingö, Sweden, 6–8 September.

Johnson, T. J. (1982) 'The state and the professions: pecularities of the British', in A. Giddens and G. Mackenzie (eds), *Social Class and the Division of Labour: Essays in Honour of Ilya Neustadt*, Cambridge: Cambridge University Press.

Kearns, G., Lee, W. R. and Rogers, J. (1989) 'The interaction of political and economic factors in the management of urban public health', in M. C. Nelson and J. Rogers (eds), *Urbanisation and the Epidemiologic Transition*, Uppsala: Meddelande från Familjehistoriska Projektet, Historiska Institutionen, Uppsala Universitet No. 9.

Kjaerheim, K. (1980) *Mellom Kloke Koner og Hvitkledde Menn: Det Norske Jordmorvesenet på 1800-tallet*, Universitetet i Oslo: Seksjon for Medisinsk Historie.

Kolberg, J. E. (ed.) (1991) *The Welfare State as Employer*, London: M. E. Sharpe.

Larsen, Ö. and Hodne, F. (1988) 'Health conditions, population and physicians in Norway 1814–1986: notes on the development of a profession', in A. Brändström and L. G. Tedebrand (eds), *Society, Health and Population during the Demographic Transition*, Stockholm: Almquist and Wiksell.

Lewis, J. (1980) *The Politics of Motherhood*, London: Croom Helm.

Martinsen, K. (1989) *Omsorg, Sykepleie og Medisin: Historisk-filosofiske Essays*, Oslo: Tano.

Maurseth, P. (1979) *Sentraladministrasjonens Historie, Bind 1, 1814–1844*, Oslo: Universitetsforlaget.

Nelson, M. C. (1992) 'När professorerna tok hand om hälsan: den tidiga hälsovårdsnämnden i Uppsala', paper presented at Nordisk Forskersymposium om Humanistisk Sundhedforskning', 4–6 March.

Nordby, T. (1987) 'Profesjokratiets periode innen norsk helsevesen – institusjoner, politikk og konfliktemner', *Historisk Tidsskrift* 3: 301–23.

—— (1989) *Karl Evang: En biografi*, Oslo: Aschehoug.

—— (1993) 'Det offentlige helsevesenet – en fagstyrets høyborg' in T. Nordby (ed.), *Arbeiderpartiet og Planstyret 1945–1965*, Oslo: Universitetsforlaget.

OECD (1987) *Financing and Delivering of Health Care*, Paris: OECD.

Parsons, T. (1964) 'Introduction', in M. Weber, *The Theory of Social and Economic Organization*, New York: Free Press.

Qvarsell, R. (1992) 'Socialmedicinen och den sociale ingeniörskonsten', paper presented at conference on 'Social Ingenjörskonst i Teori och Praktik', University of Linköping, Sweden, 9–11 June.

Riska, E. (1988) 'The professional status of physicians in the Nordic countries', *Milbank Quarterly* 66 (Suppl. 2): 133–47.
Rogers, J. and Nelson, M. C. (1989) 'Controlling infectious diseases in ports: the importance of the military in central-local relations', in M. C. Nelson and J. Rogers (eds), *Urbanisation and the Epidemiologic Transition*, Uppsala: Meddelande från Familjehistoriska Projektet, Historiska Institutionen, Uppsala Universitet No. 9.
Seip, A. L. (1984) *Sosialhjelpstaten Blir Til: Norsk Sosialpolitikk 1740–1920*, Oslo: Gyldendal.
Sommervold, W. (1993) 'Ledelse som del av svensk sykepleietradisjon', paper presented at Forum for Helsetjenesteforskning, Oslo, Norway, 30 September.
Statistisk Sentralbyrå (1978) *Historisk Statistik*, Oslo.
Statistiska Centralbyrån (1969) *Historisk Statistik för Sverige*, Stockholm.
—— (1991/2) *Hälsan i Sverige. Hälsostatistisk Årsbok*, Stockholm.
Straath, B. and Torstendahl, R. (1992) 'State theory and state development: states as network structures in change in modern European history', in R. Torstendahl (ed.), *State Theory and State History*, London: Sage.
Tengvald, K. (1988) 'Samhället och folkhälsan', in U. Himmelstrand and G. Svensson (eds), *Sverige – Vardag och Struktur. Sociologer Beskriver det Svenska Samhället*, Stockholm: Norstedts.
Therborn, G. (1989) *Borgarklass och Byråkrati i Sverige*, Lund: Arkiv.
Torstendahl, R. (1985) 'Engineers in Sweden and Britain 1829–1914: professionalisation and bureaucratisation in a comparative perspective', in W. Conze and J. Kocka (eds), *Bildungsbürgertum im 19. Jahrhundert*, Stuttgart: Klett-Cotta.
—— (1991) *Bureaucratisation in Northwestern Europe, 1880–1985: Domination and Governance*, London: Routledge.
Weir, M. and Skocpol, T. (1985) 'State structures and the possibilities for "Keynesian" responses to the Great Depression in Sweden, Britain, and the United States', in P. B. Evans, D. Rueschemeyer and T. Skocpol (eds), *Bringing the State Back In*, Cambridge: Cambridge University Press.

13 The medical profession in the Nordic countries
Medical uncertainty and gender-based work

Elianne Riska and Katarina Wegar

In the early sociological literature on the professions, doctors were portrayed as solo fee-for-service practitioners (see, for instance, Parsons 1951). This picture corresponds to that of contemporary health care delivery, which has, however, been transformed in most Western countries into a corporate or public primary-care system and a highly specialized and technology-intensive hospital system. During the past decade, this structural change in health care delivery has been the focus of a debate waged in the study of the professions. At issue has been the consequences of this change for the doctors who increasingly are practising in bureaucratic settings. Quite different views have been put forward. Some have advanced a proletarianization thesis of the gradual loss of control over work and autonomy of the medical profession as it becomes the subject of the aims and control of external corporate interests in health care (McKinlay and Arches 1985; McKinlay and Stoeckle 1988; see also Murphy 1990). Others have proposed a restratification thesis that the medical profession will be able to maintain its professional power and autonomy because it has developed an internal differentiation to counter the threats to its dominance in the medical division of labour (Freidson 1984, 1985; Ritzer and Nakzak 1988).

The two hypotheses have added important new dimensions to the literature on the medical profession. The major merit of the proletarianization thesis is that its proponents – like those of the later neo-Weberian perspective (see, for example, Larson 1977) – have brought attention to the economic and political factors that shape doctors' work. But its weakness is that it assumes that *all* doctors are subject to a devaluation of work and loss of work autonomy. Hence the structural source and consequence of the 'social transformation of doctoring' are identified, but a new differentiation, especially by gender, is not. Similarly, while the merit of the restratification thesis is that it points to the new internal differentiation of the medical profession, it does not consider gender as a stratifying principle in the new division of labour within the profession.

In most Western countries medicine is no longer an all-male profession. The rising proportion of women in this profession, especially over the past twenty years, has been the focus of research on the changing proportion of women among medical students and medical practitioners (see, for instance, Riska and Wegar 1993a). The influx of women into medicine can be attributed to broader cultural and economic forces which have changed women's position in society. In addition, in most societies three state-initiated measures have strengthened women doctors' position. First, abolishment of discriminatory practices against women and affirmative action policies have increased women's proportion among medical students. Second, the new medical schools, which were established in the 1970s, were part of a social reform movement in medicine which emphasized community medicine and primary-care education. The increased admission of medical students by the new medical schools led to an opening of medical education particularly to women (Riska 1989; Elston 1993). Third, simultaneously in some countries welfare-state policies resulted in reforms in primary-care delivery that were designed to narrow social inequity in health. This was particularly the case in two Nordic countries – Finland and Norway – where state legislation since the 1970s has changed the work conditions for general practitioners. This chapter will focus on the effect of these state policies, particularly on the gender division of labour in medicine. The gendered aspects of doctoring have more recently been the focus of sociological inquiry (see, for example, Lorber 1984, 1993; Witz 1992; Elston 1993; Riska and Wegar 1993b). This research has unravelled the structural mechanisms that hamper women's careers in the male-dominated medical profession. Meanwhile the mainstream approaches – that is, functionalist, neo-Weberian and neo-Marxist, including the recent debate on the social transformation of doctoring reviewed above – have continued to ignore the gender aspect of the profession. The mainstream approaches have given precedence to economic and technological factors and have relegated other factors, such as gender and race, to merely secondary importance, if they are recognized and there is any significance attributed to them at all (Stacey 1988; Wharton 1991). Yet, more research is needed to unravel the cultural and social processes that lead to the social construction of the gendered character of the existing medical division of labour.

This chapter approaches the gender segregation of work among doctors by examining a key element in the social construction of the power of the medical profession – the capacity to manage medical uncertainty. It is argued that the gender segregation of work is perpetuated by different claims to mastering this uncertainty. While the male-dominated areas of medicine strive to consolidate the technical and medical expertise of the profession, women doctors work mainly in areas where additional 'female' skills are used to manage medical uncertainty.

MEDICAL UNCERTAINTY AND THE POWER OF DOCTORS

The element of uncertainty and the mastery of it have been core characteristics in the social organization of medicine as a profession. Talcott Parsons recognized this feature of medicine when he suggested that 'magic beliefs and practices tend to cluster about situations where there is an important uncertainty factor and where there are strong emotional interests in the success of the action' (1951: 469). Historically viewed, professions became the agents managing the tensions and emotions involved in social situations characterized by uncertainty as this task was transferred from the domestic sphere to the market.

Although the functionalist approach recognized the segregation of tasks by gender in the domestic domain (that is to say, sex roles), market relations were depicted as gender-neutral. Parsons' pattern variables describing the professional values and professional culture shaped the thoughts of a whole generation of sociologists (Turner 1993: 14) and resulted in a normative theory of professions. The norms of the profession and the professional socialization of the aspiring members became crucial elements in explaining the status and behaviour of the medical profession in the market (Parsons 1951; Merton *et al.* 1957). Hence, medical education provides future members of the profession not only with the scientific knowledge that will enable them to master the body but also with the norms that guide professional behaviour. In the process of professional socialization, previous particularistic features that have shaped the individual's socialization and behaviour, for example gender and race, became obsolete. Neither the particularistic characteristics of the client nor those of the professional were to interfere in the professional service.

The ideal of professional neutrality has, however, been modelled after stereotypical male attributes, such as assertiveness and being in control. Particularly specialties with high prestige have been presumed to require stereotypically masculine personality traits. Lorber notes that 'both students and faculty have preconceived notions of the fit of personalities and the demands of the specialties' (1984: 32). Also in her work on the history of women's entry into the American medical profession, Walsh (1977) shows that early assumptions of the unsuitability of women for medical work were based on the premise that their feminine sensibilities in turn would make them unsuitable for medical practice. In brief, the ideal of professional 'neutrality' contains contradictions and as a professional strategy it has been used to legitimate contradictory claims.

The basis of the power of the medical profession is its claim to mastering a scientific knowledge and professing a service orientation. Yet as sociologists have amply documented, a crucial part of medical socialization consists in learning how to cope with medical uncertainty (Fox 1957; Light 1979). Recent work on the socialization of medical students confirms this central feature. In medical school and during internships, medical students internalize rules for controlling emotions and anxieties about their incomplete knowledge of how to diagnose or solve diffuse or complicated medical problems. For example, Hafferty (1988) has shown that cadaver stories are still part of the emotional socialization of medical students. In her study of medical students, Anspach (1988) pointed to the tacit function of case presentations. They enforced a reductionist view of factors influencing bodily processes: only non-human factors were depicted as determining the outcome of the disease process or the treatment, thereby relieving the physician of responsibility.

The service orientation and the altruism of the profession have not only formed crucial elements in defining the character of professions in the market (see Parsons 1951; Freidson 1970). These elements have also been part of the ideology of 'liberal medicine' (Herzlich 1982), also called the sacred trust (Harris 1969) of the medical profession. The service orientation of doctors and the ethical aspects of doctoring have been used by the medical profession in various countries to ward off the intrusion of state involvement in the market relation between the clients and the profession (see also Riska and Vinten-Johansen 1981; Vinten-Johansen and Riska 1991). In this regard, the service orientation has served as a collectivist and demarcationary strategy of the profession against the power of the state as well as other health professions. As will be shown, women doctors can use this strategy to defend the niches they at present occupy in medicine and claim them as their own against the male-dominated segments of medicine.

GENDERED WORK IN MEDICINE: MANAGING MEDICAL UNCERTAINTY

The 'feminization' of the medical profession

Since the early 1970s, in most advanced industrial countries women have entered the medical profession in growing numbers. In 1970, in the United Kingdom, for example, 26 per cent of the students entering medical schools were women; a figure that had increased to 49 per cent in 1989. At the same time, the proportion of women among active practitioners has risen from slightly less than one-fifth in 1970 to more than one-quarter in 1990 (Elston 1993). In the United States the proportion of women doctors increased from 7 per cent to 18 per cent between 1970 and 1992 and is projected to reach 30 per cent by the year 2010 (Kletke *et al.* 1990). In the Nordic countries the proportion of women doctors had reached the current Anglo-American level by 1970. The proportion is projected to increase even further in the future. By 1995, between a quarter and a half of all the doctors in the Nordic countries are expected to be women (Table 13.1). In Finland the proportion will be even higher so that a majority of the physicians will be women by year 2000.

Although the proportion of women has increased rapidly, it is not entirely adequate to portray the change as a 'feminization', as is common in current literature. Women doctors still constitute only a fifth or a third at most of the members of the medical profession, and such a proportion can hardly amount to a 'feminization' of the profession. Furthermore, so far it is rather a question of a 'ghettoization' of the women doctors within the profession than an entry as equals at all levels of the profession (Lorber 1993). The statistics from the United Kingdom, the United States and the Nordic countries give the same picture: women doctors tend more often to work in primary-care specialties than their male colleagues. Typically they are salaried and have lower incomes than men doctors (Riska and Wegar 1993b).

This gender segregation of work follows the extent of emotion work involved. Men tend to practise in settings where control of emotion is part of their job (see James 1989: 37). By contrast, women more often practise in specialties and

Table 13.1 The proportion of women in the medical profession in the Nordic countries, 1985–2025 (%)

Year	Denmark	Finland	Iceland	Norway	Sweden
1985	24	39	11	19	31
1990	26	42	16	23	34
1995	33	48	21	28	37
2000	37	52	25	31	40
2010	45	58	33	40	45
2020	56	64	45	49	51
2025	61	64	50	51	52

Source: SNAPS (1986, 1992).

settings that expose them to frequent face-to-face interactions with clients. In their practice a central part of women doctors' work is to deal with other people's vague complaints and feelings.

Emotion work has traditionally been viewed as women's work because of women's presumed 'natural' propensities for this type of work even on the labour market (Hochschild 1979; James 1989). Hearn (1982: 193) has called this feature of women's caring work 'the patriarchal feminine': it conforms to the feminine caring stereotype at the same time as it complements and reinforces the masculine stereotype. Hearn (1982: 195) views professionalization as the masculinization of the behaviour of practitioners and final domination of patriarchal values of rationality over the ideology of femininity and emotionality. Recently Witz (1992: 1–6) has advanced a similar approach in the study of professions. She points to the existence in the history of professions not only of male but also of female 'professional projects'. She argues that the female professional projects have always been constrained by and subordinated to the male professional projects that are part of the overarching patriarchal control of female labour.

Although women as carers mostly work in positions or settings where they are subordinated to men, they have managed to demarcate a territory of their own by appealing to their womanly skills. That women doctors in primary care also use this strategy is evident in a study conducted on the work of women doctors in Finland.

The social transformation of medicine: Norway and Finland

As early as the nineteenth century, access to medical care in Finland, Norway and Sweden was secured by the establishment of a public sector. The late industrialization and a rurally dispersed population in these countries did not enable the rise of a profession of independent practitioners in a free market. Instead, the modern medical profession was born within a public organization of medical practice and composed from the beginning mainly of salaried employees (Riska 1993).

Since the Second World War, two major external factors have, however, changed medical practice in the Nordic countries: first, the scientific and technological development of medicine and, second, the public expansion of primary care from 1965 to 1985. Access to a capital-intensive structure of health care, control over management positions in hospitals and close connections to physician-policy-makers representing state authorities have in fact bolstered the previous strong position of hospital physicians. The professional power and autonomy of hospital physicians have therefore changed very little in Finland, Norway and Sweden over the past century (Riska 1993).

By contrast, the position of the general practitioner has dramatically changed as increased public access to primary care was initiated as a measure of welfare state policies. Two Nordic countries – Norway and Finland – vividly illustrate this point. The Public Health Act of 1972 in Finland and the Municipal Health Act of 1984 in Norway created a new breed of doctor: the municipal health-centre doctor in Finland and the municipal doctor in Norway. Both are municipal, salaried employees. Their work is characterized by a bureaucratic setting that grants them little control over the choice and number of clients. This group of doctors fits the criteria of so-called 'welfare state occupations', that is, they derive their legitimacy from their function in the welfare state (Elzinga 1990: 162). In the case of these doctors, the positions were created to narrow social inequity in health. Between 1979 and 1988, the municipal doctors grew from 3 per cent to 41 per cent of all general practitioners in Norway (Elstad 1991a: 122). In 1993, a fifth of all doctors in Finland were working at municipal health centres (Finnish Medical Association 1993).

In addition, two other types of general practitioner coexist in Norway: the old-time independent private practitioner and a new category called contract doctor ('*avtaleleger*') (Elstad 1991b). The latter is an independent practitioner who on the basis of a contract with the municipality provides services to patients. The contract doctors, who constituted half of the general practitioners in 1989, are reimbursed by the state through the local social insurance agency, a fee-for-service system called '*styckprisrefusjon*'. This system has considerably advanced the possibility for increased incomes for this group of doctors: 42 per cent of the contract doctor's income came from this system in 1989 (Elstad 1991b: 58). A contractual basis of medical practice has, however, been shown to hamper women's entry and work in such settings both in the United Kingdom and in the United States (Elston 1993; Lorber 1993). The trend among doctors who set up group practice seems to be that women doctors' entry and terms of work in such settings are controlled by their male colleagues.

The models of providing public primary care in Finland and Norway form an interesting example of women doctors' control over work in primary care. In the case of Norway, general practitioners had already established general practice as a specialty when the Municipal Health Act was enacted in 1984. They were guaranteed clients and financial security as the positions of municipal doctor were established. By contrast, in Finland the positions of municipal health-centre doctors were created before the organization of general practice as a specialty. Doctors working in these positions need not be in a specialty.

The professionalization of general practice prior to the provision of a structure securing its practice resulted in the continuation and consolidation of a male-dominance among general practitioners in Norway. In 1993, 72 per cent of the doctors in general practice and 86 per cent of the doctors in leading administrative positions in the municipal health system were men (Den Norske Laegeforening 1993). In 1993, 25 per cent of the doctors in Norway were women as compared to 44 per cent in Finland.

In Finland, the lack of any organized group of specialists among the municipal health-centre doctors has kept this group professionally weak. Specialist status is still not required for doctors working at municipal health centres. This circumstance might be both a cause and an effect of the dominance of women doctors: by 1993, 55 per cent of the municipal health-centre doctors were women (Finnish Medical Association 1993). Thus, job opportunities in the public sector were primarily offered to non-specialized doctors. Over the past thirty years, a clear trend can be discerned in women and men doctors' tendency to gain specialty credentials. In 1960, 38 per cent of the women were specialists compared to 42 per cent of the men. In 1993, 37 per cent of the women worked as specialists, but 58 per cent of the men (Finnish Medical Association 1993).

The 'female gaze' of women doctors in primary care

Data gathered through interviews of women doctors (N = 31) in Finland in 1987 (Riska and Wegar 1993a) show that women municipal health-centre doctors are by means of a *discursive strategy* (Witz 1992: 204) legitimating their competence in this kind of work as they lack a formal competence as specialists. Three interrelated strategies were presented in the interviews.

First, these doctors depicted themselves as the historical link and continuity with the old-time community doctor of the pre-industrial society. Although that doctor was a man, he was mainly envisioned in gender-neutral and abstract terms. He represented a social institution capturing certain values of medicine perceived as lost in the current era of biomedicine. As one woman doctor reflecting on her career choice said:

> 'If I think back, then I think that I always had a certain desire to work in a small commmunity and the old idea of the community doctor, which had been in the back of my mind all the time, was something attractive.'

The municipal health-centre doctor was viewed as a repository of the traditional values of the doctor of the pre-industrial age. Although the medical knowledge of that doctor certainly was limited, it was his concern for the patient that was seen as lost in modern bureaucratic and specialized medical practice. The women doctors felt that they as women were legitimate carriers of those values. This discourse about the old-time community doctor not only was a glorification of the past but it also was recast as a female role, to legitimate the present.

Second, women doctors considered their tasks in medicine to be more holistic than men's. Women doctors' work in medicine was described as closely linked to women's life experiences and women's caring work. As one woman put it:

> 'Men tend to think about these things more narrowly. They want to believe that if we have a problem, we deal with it and get it out of the way once and for all – without taking the background [of the patient] and the totality into account, for example, in such practical issues as the patient's living conditions and life circumstances and how his or her continued care is going to be organized.'

> (Riska and Wegar 1993a: 88)

Women doctors can appeal to management and mastery of the whole array of uncertainty related to what Armstrong (1983; 1984) has called illness related to social spaces. Such illness is related to social relations and the social and cultural factors embedded in these relations. In the male-dominated segments of the medical profession, mastery of the scientific and technical knowledge and mastery of emotions constitute the core characteristics of the professional. The 'biomedical gaze' characterizes the men doctors' strength and the settings they practise in. Women doctors, especially those in primary care, can appeal to the 'female gaze' that make them experts on illnesses related to social spaces.

Third, the women doctors considered external or social recognition of their work to be less important than the guiding norm of professional success indicated. They viewed themselves as clearly less career-oriented and more genuinely service-oriented than men. Men's dominance in surgery (for instance, 92 per cent in 1993) was explained by the different notion women had of their task in medicine – different from the stereotypic male view of 'being a doctor':

> 'Something that I also believe has an impact is that women don't experience a similar pressure to practise heroic medicine like surgery. . . . The reason why women don't chose a career in surgery I believe has to do with that they don't have such a need to be recognized or to hold the healer's knife in their hand. In some way men have different reasons for studying medicine. I believe that they are more success-oriented and have a clear sense of what a successful physician is like.'

> (Riska and Wegar 1993a: 88–9)

The men's achievement orientation, the women doctors believed, detached them from the genuine concerns of the profession: service and altruistic concerns for the patient. Women doctors in public primary care were, by definition, not guided by the business orientation of the market. They could profess that they were true, altruistic servants of the patient and that they were the sole carriers of the inherent professional ethic of the medical profession.

The discursive strategy, which appealed to the legacy of the profession and its holistic and humanistic concerns, legitimated women doctors' position not only in medicine but in primary care particularly. Professionalization of medicine has so far meant an emphasis on technical skills and scientific knowledge and those values in society associated with maleness. The results indicate that an appeal to mastery of different kinds of medical uncertainty shapes the gender division of labour in the medical profession.

CONCLUSION

During the past two decades, women in most Western countries have entered medical schools in increasing numbers. In the 1990s, they will constitute a quarter to a third of the members of the medical profession in most Western countries. Yet a clear gender segregation of work among doctors can be observed today. Women tend to cluster in certain areas of medicine – primary care and child health – and may in the future dominate in geriatrics. The question this chapter has tried to answer is how this gender-based division of labour has been constructed and is reproduced. Previous work in the field has mainly pointed to structural barriers – gatekeeping mechanisms – that hamper women's career in the profession (Lorber 1984, 1993). Hence, women doctors end up in low-level jobs and specialties enjoying little prestige and remuneration.

In addition to the structural barriers, this chapter has suggested that this gender division of labour is shaped by a central characteristic of the medical profession: its claim to having mastered medical uncertainty. Atkinson and Delamont (1990: 105–6) have suggested that the power basis of the profession lies not merely in its scientific knowledge but also in the indeterminate knowledge or professional style. The professional style of the profession is characterized by the male ethic of rationality. As the early sociological literature on the medical profession suggests, the professional style of doctors can be characterized as 'affective neutrality' (Parsons 1951) or 'detached concern' (Fox 1957). The work of women doctors, however, demands other types of skills, since they address the medical uncertainty related to illnesses of social spaces. Women doctors' claims to having mastered this type of medical uncertainty can be made on the grounds that they have the additional 'female gaze'. By appealing to this 'gaze', women doctors can demarcate certain types of work as their own. The strategy demarcates their domain both from the work done by men doctors and from the 'emotional labour' of nurses.

An increasing number of scholars have stressed that narratives should not be seen as direct reflections of inner experiences or events, but that self-understanding is shaped by prevailing social and cultural norms. Wuthnow, for example, has argued that 'the product of our interviews will not be meanings, but discourses about meanings' (1987: 63). Motives should not be understood as sources of behaviour but rather as 'a concept used by people to make actions understandable to them and to others' (Gusfield 1989: 11). In a similar manner we have in this chapter analysed the women doctors' explanations of their specialty choices and orientation as part of a discursive strategy intended to legitimate their right to perform certain medical functions. While we cannot say for sure that these women doctors in their everyday work are, for example, more service-oriented than their male colleagues, it is clear that the assertion of gender-specific competence has served as an important professional strategy.

A dimension not empirically explored in our study was whether the women doctors' claims were valid. Furthermore, the women doctors' answer to such a question can only partially be illuminated by existing research in the field. As noted in the introduction, in past sociological work on the professional behaviour of doctors, gender has not been considered to be important (see Lorber 1975). Two trends seem to have changed this perception. First, some have interpreted the increasing influx of women into medical schools and the medical profession in optimistic terms. Partly on the basis of essentialistic notions of gender, they have argued that women will change the character and content of medical practice in the future (see, for instance, Altekruse and McDermott 1987: 85; Miles 1991: 157). Second, feminist criticism of sexist bias in medical diagnosis and treatment has challenged the previous sociological notion of the universalistic criteria guiding professional behaviour.

Only a few empirical studies have so far addressed all the complex aspects of this issue. Yet there seems to be enough research evidence to support the contention that women have a more empathic style of communicating with patients than do men (Martin *et al.* 1988; Meeuwesen *et al.* 1991; Roter *et al.* 1991). That this empathic attitude is also reflected in differences in the diagnosis and treatment patterns of women and men doctors has only been given scant empirical support in existing research. In their review of the twelve studies published on this topic since 1985, Mattila and Hemminki (1993) found a gender difference in the studies of the practice of American gynaecologists and obstetricians: men were more intrusive, and women were more likely to consider conservative alternatives. Studies of general practitioners in Canada provided conflicting evidence (see, for example, Maheux *et al.* 1990; Cohen *et al.* 1991) while a Dutch study of general practitioners showed gender differences in practice style (Bensing *et al.* 1993).

While specialty has been controlled for, most of these studies do not provide information on the practice setting. Women tend to practise in settings that show a selective range of patients. Hence, practice setting and type of patients have to be controlled for if any inferences are to be drawn about gender differences in doctors' medical decision-making. That the issue is a complex one is shown in a recent factorial experiment conducted with 192 American men doctors to determine the extent of non-medical influences on medical decision-making (McKinlay *et al.* 1993). It was found that the doctors' practice setting and experience and the patient's age, race and insurance status significantly influenced certain diagnoses. Hence the affective-neutrality and universalistic criteria guiding professional behaviour, questioned already by Freidson (1970), seem to belong to the Grand Theory tradition in the sociology of professions. Approaches of the middle range tend more often to confirm the particularistic character of medical practice. This particularistic feature is increasingly going to characterize the medical profession as it is differentiated by specialty, practice setting and gender. In this regard, the discursive strategies of the subgroups of the medical profession serve as a means of maintaining professional power in the prevailing medical division of labour.

REFERENCES

Altekruse, J. M. and McDermott, S. W. (1987) 'Contemporary concerns of women in medicine', in S. V. Rossner (ed.), *Feminism within the Science and Health Professions: Overcoming Resistance*, Oxford: Pergamon Press.

Anspach, R. R. (1988) 'Notes on the sociology of medical discourse: the language of case presentation', *Journal of Health and Social Behavior* 29: 357–75.

Armstrong, D. (1983) *The Political Anatomy of the Body: Medical Knowledge in Britain in the Twentieth Century*, Cambridge: Cambridge University Press.

—— (1984) 'The patient's view', *Social Science and Medicine* 18: 737–44.

Atkinson, P. and Delamont, S. (1990) 'Professions and powerlessness', *The Sociological Review* 38: 90–110.

Bensing, J. M., van den Brink-Muinen, A. and Bakker, D. H. (1993) 'Gender differences in practice style: a Dutch study of general practice', *Medical Care* 31: 219–29.

Cohen, M., Ferrier, B., Woodward C. and Goldsmith, C. (1991) 'Gender differences in practice patterns of Ontario family physicians', *Journal of the American Medical Women's Association* 46: 49–53.

Elstad, J. I. (1991a) 'En helse- og sosialarbeider? Profesjonsstrid og lagdeling i helse- og sosialsektoren', in H. Piene (ed.), *Helsevesen i Knipe: En Antologi om Helsetjenesteforskning*, Oslo: Ad Notam.

—— (1991b) *Flere Leger, Større Bruk? Artikler om Bruk av Allmenlegetjenester*, Oslo: INAS Rapport 91: 11.

Elston, M. A. (1993) 'Women doctors in a changing profession: the case of Britain', in E. Riska and K. Wegar (eds), *Gender, Work and Medicine: Women and the Medical Division of Labour*, London: Sage.

Elzinga, A. (1990) 'The knowledge aspect of professionalization: the case of science-based nursing education in Sweden', in R. Torstendahl and M. Burrage (eds), *The Formation of Professions: Knowledge, State and Strategy*, London: Sage.

Finnish Medical Association (1993) *Physicians in Finland 1993* (Abstract).

Fox, R. C. (1957) 'Training for uncertainty', in R. Merton, G. G. Reader and P. L. Kendall (eds), *The Student-Physician*, Cambridge, Mass.: Harvard University Press.

Freidson, E. (1970) *Profession of Medicine: A Study in the Sociology of Applied Knowledge*, New York: Dodd, Mead & Co.

—— (1984) 'The changing nature of professional control', *Annual Review of Sociology* 10: 1–20.

—— (1985) 'The reorganization of the medical profession', *Medical Care Review* 42: 11–35.

Gusfield, J. (ed.) (1989) *Kenneth Burke: On Symbols and Society*, Chicago: Chicago University Press.

Hafferty, F. W. (1988) 'Cadaver stories and the emotional socialization of medical students', *Journal of Health and Social Behavior* 29: 344–56.

Harris, R. (1969) *A Sacred Trust*, Baltimore: Penguin Books.

Hearn, J. (1982) 'Notes on patriarchy, professionalization and the semi-professions', *Sociology* 16: 184–202.

Herzlich, C. (1982) 'The evaluation of relations between French physicians and the state from 1880 to 1980', *Sociology of Health and Illness* 4: 241–53.

Hochschild, A. R. (1979) 'Emotion work, feeling rules and social structure', *American Journal of Sociology* 85: 551–75.

James, N. (1989) 'Emotional labour: skill and work in the social regulation of feelings', *Sociological Review* 37: 15–41.

Kletke, P. R., Marder, W. D. and Silverberger, A. B. (1990) 'The growing proportion of female physicians: implications for US physician supply', *American Journal of Public Health* 80: 300–4.

Larson, M. S. (1977) *The Rise of Professionalism*, Berkeley: University of California Press.

Light, D. W. (1979) 'Uncertainty and control in professional training', *Journal of Health and Social Behavior* 20: 310–22.
Lorber, J. (1975) 'Women and medical sociology: invisible professionals and ubiquitous patients', in M. Millman and R. Moss Kanter (eds) *Another Voice: Feminist Perspectives on Social Life and Social Science*, New York: Anchor Books.
—— (1984) *Women Physicians*, London: Tavistock.
—— (1993) 'Why women will never be true equals in the American medical profession', in E. Riska and K. Wegar (eds), *Gender, Work and Medicine: Women and the Medical Division of Labour*, London: Sage.
McKinlay, J. B. and Arches, J. (1985) 'Towards the proletarianization of physicians', *International Journal of Health Services* 15(2): 161–95.
McKinlay, J. B., Potter, D. and Feldman, H. A. (1993) 'Non-medical influences on medical decision-making', unpublished paper, New England Research Institute, Watertown, Mass.
McKinlay, J. B. and Stoeckle, J. D. (1988) 'Corporatization and the social transformation of doctoring', *International Journal of Health Services* 18(2): 191–205.
Maheux, B., Dufort, F., Belland, F. and Jaques, A. (1990) 'Female medical practitioners: more preventive and patient oriented?', *Medical Care* 28: 87–92.
Martin, S. C., Arnold, R. M. and Parker, R. (1988) 'Gender and medical socialization', *Journal of Health and Social Behavior* 29: 191–205.
Mattila, S. and Hemminki, E. (1993) 'Onko nais- ja mieslääkäreiden hoitokäytännöillä eroa', unpublished paper, Department of Public Health Science, University of Helsinki.
Meeuwesen, L., Schaap, C. and van der Staak, C. (1991) 'Verbal analysis of doctor–patient communication', *Social Science and Medicine* 32: 1143–50.
Merton, R., Reader, G. G. and Kendall, P. L. (eds) (1957) *The Student-Physician*, Cambridge, Mass.: Harvard University Press.
Miles, A. (1991) *Women, Health and Medicine*, Milton Keynes: Open University Press.
Murphy, R. (1990) 'Proletarianization or bureaucratization: the fall of the professional?', in R. Torstendahl and M. Burrage (eds), *The Formation of Professions: Knowledge, State and Strategy*, London: Sage.
Den Norske Laegeforening (1993) *1993 Legestatistikk.*
Parsons, T. (1951) *The Social System*, New York: Free Press.
Riska, E. (1989) 'Women's careers in medicine: developments in the United States and Finland', *Scandinavian Studies* 61: 185–98.
—— (1993) 'The medical profession in the Nordic countries', in F. Hafferty and J. B. McKinlay (eds), *The Changing Medical Profession: An International Perspective*, New York: Oxford University Press.
Riska, E. and Vinten-Johansen, P. (1981) 'The involvement of behavioral sciences in American medicine: a historical perspective', *International Journal of Health Services* 11: 583–96.
Riska, E. and Wegar, K. (1993a) 'Women physicians: a new force in medicine?', in E. Riska and K. Wegar (eds), *Gender, Work and Medicine: Women and the Medical Division of Labour*, London: Sage.
—— (eds) (1993b) *Gender, Work and Medicine: Women and the Medical Division of Labour*, London: Sage.
Ritzer, G. and Nakzak, D. (1988) 'Rationalization and the deprofessionalization of physicians', *Social Forces* 67: 1–22.
Roter, D., Liplein, M. and Korsgaard, A. (1991) 'Sex differences in patients' and physicians' communication during primary care medical visits', *Medical Care* 29: 1083–93.
SNAPS (Samnordisk arbetsgrupp för prognos- och specialistutbildningsfrågor) (1986) *Den Framtida Läkararbetsmarknaden i Norden.*
—— (1992) *Den Framtida Läkararbetsmarknaden i Norden*, n.p.: Caslon Press.
Stacey, M. (1988) *The Sociology of Health and Healing: A Textbook*, London: Unwin Hyman.

Turner, B. S. (1993) 'Talcott Parsons, universalism and the educational revolution: democracy versus professionalism', *British Journal of Sociology* 44: 1–24.

Vinten-Johansen, P. and Riska, E. (1991) 'New Oslerians and Real Flexnerians: the response to threatened professional autonomy', *International Journal of Health Services* 21: 75–108.

Walsh, M. R. (1977) *Doctors Wanted: No Women Need Apply: Sexual Barriers in the Medical Profession, 1835–1975*, New Haven: Yale University Press.

Wharton, A. (1991) 'Structure and agency in socialist-feminist theory', *Gender and Society* 5: 373–89.

Witz, A. (1992) *Professions and Patriarchy*, London: Routledge.

Wuthnow, R. (1987) *Meaning and Moral Order: Explorations in Cultural Analysis*, Berkeley: University of California Press.

14 Post-communist reform and the health professions
Medicine and nursing in the Czech Republic

Alena Heitlinger

INTRODUCTION

The November 1989 Velvet Revolution, which ended more than forty years of communist rule in Czechoslovakia, also brought to an end the socialist experiment in 'free' health care as both an individual civil right and a collective (that is to say, state) responsibility. Since the Velvet Revolution, pressure has been mounting to make changes in the health care system as quickly as possible, and a complete reorganization of the 'public service' model of health care is currently under way. The major goals of this chapter are (1) to explore the central features of the state socialist health care system and the proposed health care reforms; (2) to assess the significance of the communist and the post-communist state for medical and nursing prerogatives, and for the income and power of practitioners; (3) to review early experiences with health care reform implementation; and (4) to evaluate the impact of the reforms on profession–state relations.

THE DOMINANT FEATURES OF THE STATE SOCIALIST/COMMUNIST HEALTH CARE SYSTEM[1]

The role of the communist party-state in the health care system

Like its Soviet counterpart, the Czechoslovak socialist health service system was a state-operated, tax-financed, specialized branch of the general public service. The communist party-state exercised tight budgetary control over medical facilities, technologies, drugs and salaries, and a high degree of administrative power over health norms and standards. With few exceptions (for instance, the health care services for the party *nomenklatura*, the army and railway workers), the entire health service was centralized under the Czech and Slovak Ministries of Health.[2] At the top of the organizational pyramid was the so-called 'chief specialist' (a physician by training), who was a full-time administrative official of the national Ministry of Health with responsibility for medical standards. The chief specialist gave direction to the officially designated regional and district specialists. Party membership was a requirement for these positions of authority in the administration of health services, though this was usually not necessary for the more clinical work of chiefs of hospital departments and ambulatory clinics.

In theory, the officially designated specialists, especially those at the national and regional level, combined authority based on expertise with that based on office, and as such played an important role in the centralized planning of health care. However, as members of the communist *nomenklatura*, the chief specialists were more likely to defend the interests of the party-state than the professional and corporate interests of medicine. Moreover, the Czech and Slovak Ministries of Health were responsible only for setting policy on 'expert' medical issues; the actual control of personnel and organizational matters in local health care centres was left to the national committees, the municipal agencies of the state administration. Thus the Czech and Slovak Ministries of Internal Affairs, which controlled and coordinated the work of the national committees, rather than the two Ministries of Health, functioned as the senior decision-making bodies in many areas of the health care system (Pehe 1990).

The influence of the health ministries and their chief specialists was also limited by the central economic plan, over which they had no control. The central plan not only specified the overall low budget for health care services (reflecting the low priority assigned by the communist élites to the 'unproductive' service sector, which included health services), but also provided detailed spending norms within that budget. Like its Soviet counterpart, the Czechoslovak health system tended to use more of the resources that were relatively cheap – the services of doctors and 'middle-level' health workers such as nurses, physiotherapists or dental laboratory technicians – and fewer of the resources that were expensive – such as imported pharmaceuticals or sophisticated medical technology. Until quite recently, the average earnings of practising physicians in the Czech public health service were about one and a half the average wage, while physicians in private practice in Germany earned about four times the average wage (Cichon 1991: 321). Demand for many pharmaceuticals and sophisticated technology could be fully met neither by internal production nor by imports from the Western countries, resulting in substantial shortages and a highly visible health care crisis (Procházková 1990).

The public service health system worked as a 'defined income scheme',

> in which the volume and structure of services available were defined by whatever total income the public service was able to obtain from the general budget and by the ways in which resources were allocated to various categories of care in different regions.
>
> (Cichon 1991: 320)

While the state guaranteed access to medical services to all citizens irrespective of income, there was a severe restriction on the right of patients to choose their own physician. Anyone requiring medical care had to see a particular doctor in the patient's place of residence or work. Patients could switch doctors officially only if they could prove that they had received inadequate care from their assigned physician, and then only after a lengthy bureaucratic procedure.

The right to universal health care was further limited by an explicit rationing of medical services according to the state-determined priorities of industrial development and population replacement. Within the context of low overall health care expenditures (3.6 per cent of GNP in 1970; 5.4 per cent in 1988), the party élites assigned the best care to young workers in certain hazardous occupations in heavy industry (for example, mining and steel work), followed by expectant mothers and children. The singling out of young workers, expectant mothers and children as 'preferred' groups in the provision of health care helped to keep expenditures down, since these population groups are, on average, the least expensive to keep healthy. As a general rule, complicated surgical operations were simply not performed once a person reached a retirement age, with the exception of those eligible to attend the special party clinics (Heitlinger 1987: 95).

The medical profession under state socialism

Unlike the 'private' professions that have limited state involvement and employment (the American case) or the state-involved professions of Canada and Western Europe, state socialist professionals were primarily state-located and state-employed (Krause 1991). Socialist medicine was dependent on the state for overall financing, provision of the workplace, medical supplies and technology, clientele, salaries, medical education, licence to practise, and an adequate supply of subordinate health workers. The party-state decreed by fiscal and legislative/ administrative means the organizational framework of health services, who should receive them and in what order of priority. The determination of clinical practice was left largely in the hands of the professionals themselves, although the technological resources available to physicians to implement clinical decisions were severely restricted.

The medical profession had also some degree of control over medical education. Until 1977, professors at individual medical faculties were able both to design their curricula and to publish their own cyclostyled textbooks (the so-called student scripts). This form of professional autonomy was lost to the state in 1977, when the Czech Ministry of Education centralized the production of *all* university textbooks, in all academic disciplines, under a unified editorial plan. The first medical textbook published under the auspices of the Ministry of Education (which designated a group of 'prominent' university scholars as authors of the textbooks) came out in 1980; by 1985, all medical textbooks were published in this way (Jarolímek 1980, 1982). While the choice of the specific 'prominent scholars' undoubtedly involved some political considerations and did not necessarily include the best experts, the authors of the textbooks were none the less recognized members of the knowledge élite of the medical profession. The medical profession also maintained some of its economic prerogatives, despite the salaried status of physicians (and of everybody else) under the communist regime. As Freidson points out in a different context, relationship to the market is much more important than employment status:

If one's goods or services are so highly valued on the market that consumers are clamouring for access to them, then one can exercise considerable control over the terms, conditions, content and goals of one's work. . . . Given a strong position in the market, one can be employed and 'write one's own ticket' nonetheless.

(1984: 9)

State socialist economies were 'consumer-weak'. In order to obtain goods and services in short supply, or to improve their quality, consumers were frequently forced to resort to bribes. For the client, there was little difference between a physician, a car dealer or a plumber in this respect, although bribing a physician for a medically necessary treatment or life-saving drugs in short supply may be literally matter of life and death, and as such considered a high priority. Offering and accepting 'under-the-counter' payments is part of what Kemény (1982) calls the shadow market, where providers of service (that is, physicians and nurses) used gratuities to adjust their low salaries imposed by the central authorities. However, by accepting these bribes, physicians and nurses undermined one of the key claims to a professional status – the rendering of an altruistic service to the public.

Despite this less than desirable situation for citizens, medicine attained a high professional status in Czechoslovakia. Sociological studies on rank ordering of occupations, conducted in the 1960s and early 1990s, revealed a high occupational prestige for medicine, as high as in the United States (Heitlinger 1991; Tuček 1993). However, because of the Communist Party's insistence on a monopoly of power and doctrine, an independent medical profession free of party control could not emerge to campaign for higher salaries and better provision of medical technology. Thus, high professional status did not translate into corporate political power.

Nursing under state socialism

Czechoslovak nursing during the communist period did not fit any of the defining characteristics of a profession. Czech nurses had virtually no professional status, autonomy or prestige, and their official income was well below the average industrial wage. Doctors tended to regard nurses as 'subordinates implementing their will rather than as co-workers' and communication between the two occupational groups was generally poor (Heitlinger 1987: 121). Nurses belonged to the category of 'middle-level' health care workers. The term 'middle-level' reflected an occupational requirement for a 'middle-level' vocational education, which was acquired at specialized four-year nursing high schools. Thus most aspiring nurses entered training at the very young age of 15, when they had to choose among three primary care nursing specializations: general, paediatric and obstetrics/gynaecology. While most practising nurses were not restricted to these three specialties, a district women's nurse or labour and delivery nurse had to be formally qualified as a women's nurse.[3] Similarly, nurses employed at neonatal intensive care units had to be specialized paediatric nurses, as did teachers in childcare facilities (Heitlinger 1987: 112–13).

The comparatively low 'middle-level' educational requirement and the limited emphasis on the psycho-social needs of patients (manifested both in nursing education and in clinical practice) made it hard for nurses to emphasize any special qualities, knowledge or skills that they had and physicians lacked. Even the traditional claim to 'nursing care' (in contrast to the medical claim to 'cure') was problematic, because much of the work nurses actually performed was quite menial. Sociological research conducted in fourteen randomly selected hospitals in the early 1970s revealed that nurses devoted 56 per cent of worktime to 'basic care' (that is, making beds, helping with personal hygiene and so on), 17 per cent to documentation, 5 per cent to other activities and only 22 per cent to 'specialized nursing care' involving technical expertise beyond the juris-diction of outsiders.

There is even evidence suggesting the indifference of some nurses (and of some physicians) to the needs and suffering of patients (Kříž 1991; Uzel 1992). Other critics have noted the poor quality of many childcare facilities, manifested in high child/carer ratios, excessive regimentation and authoritarian and im-personal attitudes toward children on the part of the staff – trained paediatric nurses (Heitlinger 1993b: 98). However, other anecdotal evidence suggests that there were numerous nurses who took humanitarian care seriously, who loved nursing and provided quality service in spite of financial hardship and social debasing. As Blanka Misconiová (n.d.), the first Chief Nurse of the Czech Republic, puts it, many nurses

> helped ill and powerless people without a word, trying to maintain profes-sional pride, a level of care comparable to the European standard, and continuing self-education. Foreign literature was desperately needed and sought as a means to overcome our professional isolation once our borders were shut to the West.

Like the medical–state relation, the nursing–state interface was shaped by the high degree of party-state control over the careers of experts and professionals, and by the specifics of gender. Virtually all Czech nurses were women, and their career aspirations were generally low. Despite the fact that most women were gainfully employed during the communist period, the dominant model was that of 'wife/mother with a job rather than a woman in a responsible position with a family' (Heitlinger 1987: 55). As Havelková argues,

> [The] family represented for the woman, much more than the man, the possibility of choice and escape from political blackmail. Women consciously made use of this opportunity. . . . Political blackmail usually took the form of linking professional advancement with joining the Communist Party. The number of female party members was conspicously low in comparison to male. Women opted for motherhood, and children provided an 'excuse' to not join the party even after the mother resumed employment. Women just

deliberately gave up the chance for any greater job advancement. . . . Because women gave up participation in management, they did not have their lobby in it, and their managers did not defend their interests. This further deepened the masculine character of the power and management structures, which in turn made it difficult for women to adapt themselves to the standard masculine career patterns.[4]

(1993: 69–70)

Thus there were neither ideological predispositions nor political opportunities for the professionalization of nursing. Like physicians, nurses now have greater opportunities than during the communist period to articulate their interests and engage in autonomous politics on issues that concern them. As we shall see below, both nurses and physicians are taking advantage of these new opportunities.

POST-COMMUNIST AGENDA FOR HEALTH CARE REFORM: THE PROPOSAL FOR THE REFORM OF HEALTH CARE

Civic Forum, the Czech political grouping that in November 1989 toppled the communist regime, made health a high priority issue for reform. In early January 1990, the Civic Forum's programme committee of health care workers (composed largely of physicians) published a document entitled *Principles of Health Care Reform in Czechoslovakia*. The Principles were highly critical of the state socialist health care system, and advocated major reforms (Potůček 1991). The document was published in the health weekly *Zdravotnické noviny*, which, like other newspapers, was by then free from communist control and censorship. The Principles were accompanied by a questionnaire asking readers whether or not they approved of the proposed reforms. Readers were also encouraged to respond directly, by sending letters with suggestions to the Czech Ministry of Health, which by then had a new Minister, a new advisory Scientific Council, and several new committees, including the forty-five member Working Group for Reform of the Organization of Health Care. Members of the Working Group – physicians, lawyers, economists, dentists, sociologists and other credentialed professionals – were nominated by individual branches of Civic Forum. There were twenty-five physicians on the committee (55 per cent), but neither nurses nor ordinary 'lay' consumers were included.

The Working Group revised the Principles and in May 1990 published a new consultative document, *Reform of Health Care in the Czech Republic* (Ministry of Health and Social Affairs 1990). It offered several alternative strategies for reform, and invited individual and institutional responses from both lay citizens and health care professionals. The document was also submitted for external appraisal to France, Britain and the Copenhagen-based European Section of the World Health Organization. At the conclusion of these discussions in October 1990, the final version of the document *Draft of a New System of Health Care* was submitted to the Czech Parliament (Ministry of Health 1990). The last document was approved by the Czech government as the basis for implementation of the new health care system at the end of 1990 (Potůček 1991). All three consecutive documents advocated a shift from disease and cure to health and prevention, greater individual responsibility for health, a compulsory national health insurance programme, privatization of health services and the pharmaceutical industry, patients' right to choose their own physicians, a more decentralized and pluralistic delivery and financing of health services and medical education, some minor modifications in the organization of primary care, integration of health and social services, greater humanization and increased standards of psychiatry, higher salaries for health care practitioners, an independent self-governing professional medical association, and professional (as opposed to political) control over the content of medical education and research. The *Reform of Health Care in the Czech Republic* document promoted a two-tier health system, whereby all citizens were to have access to 'standard' care covered by medical insurance; an additional 'above-standard' form of care was to be made available through private medical services, paid for directly, by purchasing additional insurance or by contributions from municipalities, employers and charities. In order to avoid major disruption in the functioning of the current health care system, it was proposed that the various reforms would be phased in stages over a period of three to four years, to be fully completed by 1995 (Ministry of Health and Social Affairs 1990).

Mandatory health insurance emerged as the key idea of the health care reform. It was seen as a multi-functional instrument which could increase the resources for health services, and at the same time improve their quality and efficiency. Various forms of health insurance financing – state, sectoral, private, capitation, fee-for-service, diagnosis related groups or some combination of these – were suggested in response to the *Reform of Health Care in the Czech Republic* proposal. While all were based on the twin principles of 'money following the patient' and 'the necessary state guarantee', no clear conception of health insurance emerged (Potůček 1993).

IMPLEMENTING THE HEALTH CARE REFORMS

The role of the post-communist state

The break up of longstanding party-state control was initiated in March 1990 by the recall of all Directors of the so-called Institutes of National Health; their positions were later refilled on a competitive basis. A whole administrative level of the organizational pyramid, the regional institutes of health (*KÚNZ – Krajský ústav národního zdraví*), was abolished by the end of the year, along with the positions of regional and district 'chief specialist' (Pehe 1990: 23). The new Civic Forum government (elected in June 1990) also closed the special party and military clinics (known as *Sanops*). During the two years it was in office, Civic Forum approved an important document about health promotion, passed a series of enabling laws for the new national health insurance system and for private medical practice, and initiated the transfer of property rights concerning hospitals and polyclinics from the central government to local governments, churches, non-profit organizations and private group and individual health care practices (in that order).

The June 1992 general elections revealed profound and, as it turned out, irreconcilable differences between Czech and Slovak approaches towards economic, social and constitutional reforms. On 1 January 1993, the country was peacefully divided into two independent states – the Czech Republic and Slovakia. Elected on a platform advocating rapid moves towards a free market economy, the new Czech government made large-scale privatization of property in all sectors of the economy, including health care, its top priority. Rather than viewing privatization as merely one instrument in a broader framework of coordinated reform measures, the Klaus government began to see privatization as the ultimate goal of the health care reform (Potůček 1993). None the less, the legal-administrative framework of the privatization process has remained under the control of the central authorities, as has, to date, the allocation of the total resources available to health care.

The national health insurance programme and the medical profession

As we noted, mandatory health insurance emerged as the key idea of the health care reform. Various forms of health insurance were suggested, but in the end the reformers picked a fee-for-service scheme covering all types of health services (including dental care), facilities and prescription drugs. An experimental 'simulated' national health insurance programme was introduced in January 1992. During the first year of its operation, the General Health Insurance Office (*Všeobecná zdravotní pojištovna*) was fully financed out of the state budget. Financing by social insurance contributions was introduced one year later to coincide with new tax and social security legislation and the peaceful break-up of Czechoslovakia into two separate countries.

The Czech insurance scheme has a fee-schedule for approximately 4,500 eligible diagnostic and therapeutic services provided to patients. Rather than attaching different amounts of money to each item on the fee schedule (as is the case in Canada), the Czech health insurance programme assigns different numbers of points, the cash value of which is calculated every four months. The points for all medical services billed by individual doctors or provider units are added up to see how many points each has 'earned'. A primary care physician typically 'earns' 55,000 points a month for his/her provider unit (Kolomacká 1992). The points 'earned' by all physicians and provider units in the country are then aggregated and the total is divided by the money available from insurance contributions to arrive at the cash value of a single point. Once this is known, doctors can be paid. In the third quarter of 1992, a point was worth 0.45 crowns, but in the last quarter of 1992 it declined to 0.34 crowns, though it remained 0.45 crowns for physicians in private practice (Holub and Zamboch 1993).

The scheme has been criticized as unnessarily complex and fiscally unrealistic, especially for hospitals and other provider units with high (and rising) overhead costs (Pavlová 1992). Like all fee-for-service schemes, physicians who perform the most services receive the most money. Since the General Health Insurance Company has a fixed budget determined by the Ministry of Finance, the more services performed, the lower the value of each point. This creates a vicious circle, because the unrealistically low cash value of each point encourages physicians to render more services in order to earn more points and higher incomes. The scheme totally ignores illness prevention, creates an enormous amount of paperwork (only some of which is computerized) and encourages cheating and deficit-financing. By chanelling up to 92 per cent of all fiscal resources for health care through the General Insurance Company, the scheme involves the same monopolistic, 'dictatorial' control over health care providers as that exercised by the communist party-state (Bošková 1993; Daňhová 1993b; Riebauerová 1993). The Ministry of Health is currently reviewing the payment system, along with the 'standard' services covered by the scheme (Holub and Zamboch 1993; JOL 1993; Justice 1993; Lom 1993).

By maintaining control over the sum total of financial resources available to the health services, the central government has kept overall health care spending relatively low. In 1991, Czechoslovakia spent 5.9 per cent of its national income on health care, compared to 5.4 per cent in 1988 (Simons 1992). Until this share is increased closer to the European average of 7.7 per cent, and until a more sensible financing of health care is adopted, average incomes of physicians (and of nurses) will remain depressed.

The privatization of medical services

While the *Reform of Health Care in the Czech Republic* viewed privatization as merely one instrument in a broader framework of coordinated reform measures, the Klaus government regards full privatization as the main goal of the health care reform. Privatization procedures are the same for health facilities and medical services as they are for any other business. Passed in 1990, the privatization regulations allow clinics, hospitals and practitioners (including nurses) to go private if they have proper licensing, the means to secure appropriate equipment and office space and the approval of three separate government committees. The government has divided health facilities into three categories: those that should not be privatized; those that should be privatized with no restrictions concerning their future use; and those that have to preserve capacity for basic health services for ten years after their privatization. The criteria for sorting health facilities into these three categories were not published, thus leaving room for arbitrary and highly politicized decisions (Potůček 1993: 9). Moreover, given the wide-ranging definition of health, 'preserving capacity for basic health services' can be interpreted very broadly, from maintaining an expensive-to-run hospital to transforming it into a much cheaper 'health massage' establishment or a warehouse for pharmaceuticals. It is also not clear how the ten-year re- striction will be enforced should the privatized facility go bankrupt, or what will happen to the national health care network when the ten-year period expires. There are well-founded fears that under the current health insurance scheme, most privatized hospitals will soon run out of money and close down (Holub and Zamboch 1993; Justice 1993).

Advocates of rapid privatization (for the most part young male doctors, large sections of the general public and the governing coalition of right-wing parties) see market competition as a way of raising health care standards and increasing individual freedom of choice. More than 600 applications were filed in 1992 by doctors and clinics hoping to go private – too many, according to critics. As with hospitals, the main worry is that private clinics and medical practices will not survive the rigours of a free market economy (Justice 1993). Other critics have noted the government's ideological preference for the submission model of privatization at the expense of a coordinated planning approach. While the government's opposition to central planning is in keeping with the post-communist emphasis on devolutionary decision-making, the submission model greatly disadvantages those who lack the skills and resources to write complex privatization proposals. Moreover, the sum total of individual submissions is unlikely to be adequately representative of regions and medical specialties. An uncoordinated approach to privatization based on individual submissions thus could totally destroy the regional integrity of the health system, a system that would be very costly to put back together should privatization fail. There is also the danger that, in the absence of a clear definition of a 'standard' health care, privatization will accelerate the drift towards an American-style two-tiered health care system that will provide quality care only for the wealthy (Šlanger 1992; Český helsinský výbor 1993; Justice 1993). The counterargument of the Ministry of Health and the Medical Chamber is that because of a substantial nationwide excess of hospitals and physicians, closure of some facilities will not jeopardize the regional integrity of the health system. Should some serious regional gaps emerge, they could be quickly filled by new, more progressive facilities and services (Hořejší 1993; interview, Ministry of Health, May 1993).

The corporate power of professional medicine

The three health care reform documents envisaged a powerful self-governing medical association, with wide-ranging legal powers and considerable professional and political influence. The Medical Chamber was expected to produce guidelines to govern medical education and clinical practice, formulate standards for evaluating professional performance, respond through disciplinary boards to consumer complaints, act as an employer, engage in fee negotiations with the national health insurance programme, lobby Parliament and the Ministry of Health, and also perform some other unspecified functions.

The legislation reinstating the self-governing Medical Chamber (after its abolition by the communist authorities in the 1950s) was passed in May 1991 following intensive lobbying by the Union of Czech Physicians. The Union was founded shortly after the Velvet Revolution as a successor organization to the short-lived Union of Czechoslovak Physicians established during the 'Prague Spring' in 1968. Adhering to proposals outlined in the three health care documents, the Medical Chamber was created as an independent self-governing body with broad educational, licensing, disciplinary, fee-bargaining and lobbying functions. The Medical Chamber is not a trade union, but the bulk of its activities has so far focused on collective bargaining. The first fee-schedule of the General Health Insurance Company was prepared in cooperation with the leaders of the Medical Chamber, but the sum total of fiscal resources available for medical services was determined by the state (Hořejší 1993). The ensuing bargaining with various agencies of the state (that is, the General Health Insurance Company, Ministry of Health, Ministry of Finance and even President Havel) over the medical payment system has overshadowed all the other functions of the Chamber. One of the reasons for the Medical Chamber's support of the government's drive towards full privatization is that market competition is regarded by the medical leadership as a promising lever with which to break-up the continuing state monopoly over health care financing and delivery (Daňhová 1993a; Hořejší 1993).

According to Potůček, the Medical Chamber, the Chamber of Dentists, the Union of Czech Physicians and the Union of Health Workers 'formed the most influential bodies engaged in public debate about the health care reform and in the creation and implementation of a new health policy, opposing some of the proposals and decisions made by the Ministry of Health' (1993: 6). However, both the Medical Chamber and the trade unions have failed spectacularly as economic lobbies. For example, at the end of 1993, the average medical salary was only 7,000 crowns a month. In contrast, the average monthly salary of Prague metro drivers was 12,000 crowns, 71 per cent higher (Daňhová 1993a). The inability of the medical lobbies to improve physicians' incomes significantly is illustrative of the limitations of the corporate power of organized medicine *vis-à-vis* the post-communist state.

The professionalization of nursing

Nursing reforms developed in parallel with medical reforms, but independently of the three health care reform documents. The nursing reform process has been shaped by a close inderdependent relationship between nursing activists and state officials. Soon after the Velvet Revolution, nurses active in the work of Civic Forum founded Nurse Clubs, which attracted 14,000 members. The Clubs were eventually transformed into a new professional organization – the Czech Association of Nurses. The Association has evolved into a credible, self-governing professional body with educational, licensing and lobbying functions. It has developed close links with the Union of Czech Physicians, the Medical Chamber, the Parliamentary Committee for Health and Social Policy and, above all, the Chief Nurse at the Ministry of Health (Daňhová 1993c, Wagnerová 1993).

The administrative position of Chief Nurse, established by the Civic Forum Minister of Health, Dr Martin Bojar, combines policy development/coordinating roles with consultative functions. So far, the Chief Nurse's job has consisted of regular meetings with nurses from all regions of the Czech Republic, and the preparation of new legislation on nursing education, job descriptions of various categories of middle-level and auxiliary health care workers, fee-schedules for nursing services within the national health insurance programme and the privatization of nursing (interviews, Ministry of Health, June 1992, May 1993).

The nursing reforms advocated by the Czech Association of Nurses and the Ministry of Health have been based on 'classic' strategies of professionalization: (1) increased educational requirements (from high school to post-secondary and university credentials); (2) formation of an independent professional 'chamber' to handle questions of nursing standards, professional development, licensing for private practice and the disciplining of members; and (3) attempts to carve out a body of skills and knowledge that would be distinct from that used by other health care workers. Foreign experts hired by the Czech Ministry of Health have advocated as priorities the upgrading of educational requirements, expanded professional autonomy, and a more client- and team-oriented approach to nursing care (interview, Ministry of Health, May 1991).

Educational reform is proceeding at a rapid pace. The 1993–4 academic year was the final opportunity for students as young as 15 to enter nursing training. The minimum age of entry has been increased from 15 to 18, and four-year nursing high schools are being converted into two-year post-secondary nursing colleges. Three new nursing programmes have been established at universities, although university graduates will not automatically be entitled to higher salaries. The early three-fold specialization into general, women's and paediatric nursing has been abolished – all nurses now have to become general nurses before they can specialize. Both the Czech Association of Nurses and the Ministry of Health have put special emphasis on professional self-development and continuing education. To this end, several new training centres offering specialized post-graduate courses on various aspects of nursing theory, clinical practice and management have been established throughout the Czech Republic (Staňková 1991; Misconiová 1992; Tigermanová 1992).

The Czech Parliament has so far resisted the creation of a Nursing Chamber on the grounds that no such body existed before the war and that there is no real need for it. Government officials and the leaders of the Czech Association of Nurses are hopeful that all-encompassing legislation about professional colleges will be passed by the end of 1993 or 1994, and that it will enable nurses to establish their own professional college. Such a college would take over many of the functions currently performed by the Czech Association of Nurses. It would focus on licensing and disciplinary functions, leaving collective bargaining to the well-regarded Union of Health Workers or the Moravian-based Union of Nurses, which has been so far largely inactive (interview, Czech Association of Nurses, May 1993).

In the short run, some nurses are facing unemployment, especially new graduates and those previously employed in health administration, paediatric and childcare facilities. Many of the latter are closing down (Mazáčová 1991;

Staňková 1991). The situation is more serious in small towns than in the country's capital. At the same time, however, several Prague nurses are leaving nursing voluntarily for much better paid unskilled jobs in the expanding tourist industry, thus creating a nursing shortage in many hospitals (interview, Ministry of Health, May 1993). The long-term prospects for nursing appear quite promising. Better integration of health and social services, and the reorientation from cure to prevention and from hospital to community and home care, may open up new employment opportunities for nurses, which would be professionally quite rewarding (Mazáčová 1991). Jaroslav Kořán, the former mayor of Prague, said in an interview that only 30 per cent of all hospital beds in Prague are filled by patients requiring short-term acute clinical care. The other 70 per cent are occupied by the chronically ill, who could be easily looked after elsewhere by nurses (Pehe 1990: 22). As a necessary 'standard' care, private nursing home care is currently covered by the national health insurance scheme.

The extent to which privatization of nursing services will alter the nursing–client relationship is hard to predict at this time. Novel job opportunities for nurses involved in primary and preventive care may be a boost for professionalization, but the move towards privatization may, in fact, hamper altruistic care. Much will depend on how many of the new nursing services will be covered by the national health insurance scheme, and how many clients can afford the extra payments required for services deemed 'above standard'.

CONCLUSION

We have seen that medicine and nursing under state socialism were *de facto* specialized branches of a poorly funded general public service. Since the November 1989 Velvet Revolution, which peacefully ended the Communist Party monopoly of power and doctrine, the health professions, especially medicine, have played an important role in setting new priorities and redesigning the existing health care system. However, state officials have retained overall control over the implementation of the health care reforms. As we noted, the Klaus government significantly altered the scope of privatization envisaged by the three consecutive health care reform documents. Rather than viewing privatization as merely one instrument in a broader framework of coordinated reform measures, it is now seen as the ultimate goal of the health care reform. However, the legal-administrative framework of the privatization process has remained under the control of the central authorities, as has the sum total fiscal resources available for health care. Early experiences with the post-communist health care reforms therefore indicate that, while health professionals have become more visible in the policy process, the state has retained its dominant role in the profession–state relation.

ACKNOWLEDGEMENTS

Research for this chapter was carried out with the assistance of grants from Trent

University and the Social Sciences and Humanities Research Council of Canada. I would like to thank Cecilia Benoit for her helpful comments on an earlier draft of this chapter.

NOTES

1 Parts of this and the subsequent section are derived from Heitlinger (1993a).
2 Prior to 1969, when Czechoslovakia became a federal republic, there was only one national Ministry of Health.
3 Midwifery was defined as a specialty of nursing rather than as an independent health occupation.
4 Lower professional achievement was also evident among women doctors, who comprise 52 per cent of all physicians. Sociological research conducted in the early 1970s revealed that Slovak women doctors spent at most two hours daily on further study, while their male colleagues could afford at least three hours a day. Thirty-one per cent of Slovak male doctors but only 10 per cent of female doctors acquired a specialist qualification (the first and second degree *atestace*) at the expected age of 34. Twenty-five per cent of Slovak women doctors did not obtain the second degree qualification because of domestic responsibilities. What this meant was that a disproportionate number of women were found among primary care physicians, for whom the second degree *atestace* was not required (Heitlinger 1991).

REFERENCES

Bošková, V. (1993) 'Jak to vidí Martin Bojar', *Zdravotnické noviny* 62: 11.
Český helsinský výbor (1993) 'Stanovisko k privatizaci zdravotnických zařízení', *Zdravotnické noviny* 62: 20.
Cichon, M. (1991) 'Health sector reforms in Central and Eastern Europe: paradigm reversed?', *International Labour Review* 130: 311–27.
Daňhová, J. (1993a) 'Naší povinností je udržet úroveň léčebné péče. Rozhovor s doc. Mudr. Bohuslavem Svobodou, CSc., prezidentem České lékařské komory, na téma české zdravotnictví dnes, vícezdrojové financování, stávka, ale nejen o tom', *Zdravotnické noviny* 62: 17.
—— (1993b) 'Bude bod 25 haléřů? Rozhovor s poslancem Mudr. Miroslavem Čerbákem, viceprezidentem České lékařské komory', *Zdravotnické noviny* 62: 17.
—— (1993c) 'Komora sester', *Zdravotnické noviny* 62: 11.
Freidson, E. (1984) 'The changing nature of professional control', *American Review of Sociology* 10: 1–20.
Havelková, H. (1993) 'A few pre-feminist thoughts', in N. Funk and M. Mueller (eds), *Gender Politics and Post-Communism: Reflections from Eastern Europe and the Former Soviet Union*, London: Routledge.
Heitlinger, A. (1987) *Reproduction, Medicine and the Socialist State*, London: Macmillan/St Martin's Press.
—— (1991) 'Hierarchy of status and prestige within the medical profession in Czechoslovakia', in A. T. Jones (ed.), *Professions and the State: Expertise and Autonomy in the Soviet Union and Eastern Europe*, Philadelphia: Temple University Press.
—— (1993a) 'The medical profession in Czechoslovakia: legacies of state socialism, prospects for the capitalist future', in F. W. Hafferty and J. B. McKinlay (eds), *The Changing Character of the Medical Profession: An International Perspective*, Oxford: Oxford University Press.
—— (1993b) 'The impact of the transition from communism on the status of women in

the Czech and Slovak Republics', in N. Funk and M. Mueller (eds), *Gender Politics and Post-Communism: Reflections from Eastern Europe and the Former Soviet Union*, London: Routledge.

Holub, P. and Zamboch, J. (1993) 'První na řadě: privatizace zdravotnictví začala v Sokolově', *Respekt* 19–25 April.

Hořejší, T. (1993) 'Lékaři se mafie nebojí', *Respekt* 10–16 May.

Jarolímek, I. (1980) 'Obsahová přestavba lékařského studia', *Československé zdravotnictví* 28: 431–4.

—— (1982) 'Učebnice pro lékařské fakulty a zásady jejich tvorby', *Československé zdravotnictví* 30: 39–42.

JOL (1993) 'Názory pana ministra', *Statim* 2: 8.

Justice, G. (1993) 'Doctors unsure market is prescription', *The Prague Post* 3–9 February.

Kemény, I. (1982) 'The unregistered economy in Hungary', *Soviet Studies* 34: 349–66.

Kolomacká, M. (1992) 'U pokladny stál: nebudou léčit jen samoplátce?', *Lidové noviny* 28 June.

Krause, E. (1991) 'Professions and the state in the Soviet Union and Eastern Europe: theoretical Issues', in A. T. Jones (ed.), *Professions and the State: Expertise and Autonomy in the Soviet Union and Eastern Europe*, Philadelphia: Temple University Press.

Kříž, J. (1991) 'Umírání za dlouhého dne', *Lidové noviny* 29 April.

Lom, P. (1993) 'Petr Lom k současným problémům zdravotnické transformace (I)', *Zdravotnické noviny* 62: 19.

Mazáčová, M. (1991) 'Sester jako kvítí: hovoříme s hlavní sestrou MZČR Blankou Misconiovou', *Večerní Praha*, 15 May.

Ministry of Health, Czech Republic (1990) *Reform of Health Care in the Czech Republic. Version II. Draft of a New System of Health Care*, Prague: Ministry of Health.

Ministry of Health and Social Affairs, Czech Republic, Working Group for the Reform (1990) *Reform of Health Care in the Czech Republic*, Prague: Ministry of Health and Social Affairs.

Misconiová, B. (n.d.) 'The position of nurses in the Czech Republic: past, present, and future', unpublished manuscript.

—— (1992) 'Healing a sick society', *World Health* September–October: 4–5.

Pavlová, A. (1992) '"Na pojišťovnu si jen hrajeme": docent Dungl navrhuje použít rakouský systém', *Mladá fronta dnes* 17 June.

Pehe, J. (1990) 'Changes in the health care system', *Report on Eastern Europe, Radio Free Europe*, 14 September.

Potůček, M. (1991) 'The health care reform in Czechoslovakia after 17 November 1989', *Journal of Public Health Medicine* 13: 290–4.

—— (1993) 'Current social policy developments in the Czech Republic – the case of health services', unpublished manuscript.

Procházková, P. (1990) 'Iluze bezplatného zdravotnictví', *Lidové noviny* 5 June.

Riebauerová, M. (1993) 'Pacient v bodovém kruhu', *Lidové noviny* 18 May.

Simons, M. (1992) 'Health care free no more', *The Globe and Mail* 17 December.

Šlanger, J. (1992) 'Kritika dosavadního postupu a současného stavu transformace zdravotnictví v České republice', unpublished manuscript.

Staňková, M. (1991) 'Připravujeme reformu zdravotnického školství', *Sestra* 1: 1.

Tigermanová, N. (1992) 'Humánní ošertovatelství v Československu', *Sestra* 2: 3.

Tuček, M. (1993) 'Jakou máme váznost mezi obecným lidem? O prestiži povoláni zvláště pak vědeckých pracovníků', *Sociologicke aktuality* 2: 14–15.

Uzel, R. (1992) 'Co nám chybí', *Lidové noviny* 5 December.

Wagnerová, R. (1993) 'Bilance ČASu (Česká asociace sester)', unpublished manuscript.

Author index

Subject index

Coláiste na hOllscoile Gaillimh

3 1111 40001 0847